Mental Health in Historical Perspective

Series Editors
Catharine Coleborne
School of Humanities and Social Science
University of Newcastle
Callaghan, NSW, Australia

Matthew Smith
Centre for the Social History of Health and Healthcare
University of Strathclyde
Glasgow, UK

Covering all historical periods and geographical contexts, the series explores how mental illness has been understood, experienced, diagnosed, treated and contested. It will publish works that engage actively with contemporary debates related to mental health and, as such, will be of interest not only to historians, but also mental health professionals, patients and policy makers. With its focus on mental health, rather than just psychiatry, the series will endeavour to provide more patient-centred histories. Although this has long been an aim of health historians, it has not been realised, and this series aims to change that.

The scope of the series is kept as broad as possible to attract good quality proposals about all aspects of the history of mental health from all periods. The series emphasises interdisciplinary approaches to the field of study, and encourages short titles, longer works, collections, and titles which stretch the boundaries of academic publishing in new ways.

More information about this series at
http://www.palgrave.com/gp/series/14806

Steven J. Taylor · Alice Brumby
Editors

Healthy Minds in the Twentieth Century

In and Beyond the Asylum

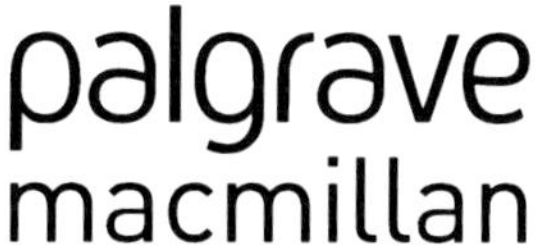

Editors
Steven J. Taylor
School of History
University of Leicester
Leicester, UK

Alice Brumby
School of Humanities, Religion and Philosophy
York St John University
York, UK

Mental Health in Historical Perspective
ISBN 978-3-030-27274-6 ISBN 978-3-030-27275-3 (eBook)
https://doi.org/10.1007/978-3-030-27275-3

This Palgrave Macmillan imprint is published by the registered company Springer Nature Switzerland AG
The registered company address is: Gewerbestrasse 11, 6330 Cham, Switzerland

Contents

Notes on Contributors

Dr. Alice Brumby is a lecturer at York St John University. Her research interests focus upon nineteenth- and twentieth-century mental health care and patient welfare in England. Her work examines the role of the community, families and patients with regard to accessing care and treatment. She has published work in *First World War Studies* and *History Today* amongst other publications. Her AHRC-funded Ph.D. examined attempts to reform mental health care. This work has contributed to a programme of public engagement, including co-curating an exhibition on the medical impact of war, in connection with the Thackray Medical Museum. She has also created exhibitions at the York Army Museum and the medical museums in Worcestershire.

Prof. Erika Dyck is a professor at the University of Saskatchewan, and a Tier 2 Canada Research Chair in the History of Medicine. She is the author of *Psychedelic Psychiatry: LSD from Clinic to Campus* (Johns Hopkins, 2008; University of Manitoba Press, 2011), *Facing Eugenics: Reproduction, Sterilization and the Politics of Choice* (University of Toronto, 2013), and *Managing Madness: The Weyburn Mental Hospital and Transformations of Psychiatric Care in Canada* (2017). She is the co-editor of the *Canadian Bulletin for Medical History*; a contributing editor to ActiveHistory.ca and a founding member of both www.historyofmadness.ca and www.eugenicsarchive.ca. In 2015, she was inducted to Canada's Royal Society in the College of New Scholars, Artists and Scientists.

Dr. Rachel Hewitt is a researcher in the history of medicine and social policy, specialising in the history of epilepsy in the late nineteenth and early twentieth centuries. Her research interests include adult and child services, labour policy, poverty and public health.

Andy Holroyde is a final-year doctoral candidate in history at the University of Huddersfield. His Ph.D. is an AHRC-funded project with the *Heritage Consortium*, examining sheltered employment and disability in the British Welfare State.

Dr. Nikki Kiyimba works as a senior lecturer in psychological trauma at the University of Chester. She also works in private practice as a Clinical Psychologist in the north-west of England. Her research interests are in using discourse analytic approaches to understanding adult and child interactions in mental health settings, and in critically evaluating constructs of psychological trauma and the mental health sequelae of traumatic and adverse events.

Dr. Jessica Lester is an associate professor of inquiry methodology (qualitative methodologies/methods) in the School of Education at Indiana University, Bloomington. Jessica's research has focused on discourse and conversation analysis, disability studies and more general concerns related to qualitative research. She is a founding member of the Microanalysis of Online Data international network and the Associate Director of the Conversation Analysis Research in Autism group.

Dr. Alice Mauger is a postdoctoral research fellow at the Centre for the History of Medicine in Ireland, School of History, University College Dublin. Her research and teaching interests include the histories of medicine, mental illness, psychiatry, alcohol and drugs in the nineteenth and twentieth centuries. Her current research project, 'Alcohol Medicine and Irish Society, c. 1890–1970' is funded by the Wellcome Trust. She has published on the history of psychiatry in Ireland, including *The Cost of Insanity in Nineteenth-Century Ireland: Public, Voluntary and Private Asylum Care* (Palgrave Macmillan, 2017).

Dr. Rob Mayo has previously worked on the conceptualisation and depiction of depression and other dysphoric conditions in David Foster Wallace's fiction and is currently working on his first book on this topic. His essay here reflects a career-long interest in science fiction, and the first steps in a new project on the theme of the mind and mental disorder in SF texts in literature, cinema and video games. He has also worked on Philip K. Dick, Daniel Keyes and Twin Peaks.

Dr Michelle O'Reilly works as an associate professor of communication in mental health at the University of Leicester. She is also a Research Consultant with Leicestershire Partnership NHS Trust. Michelle's research interests are in the language of mental health, specialising in discourse and conversation analysis. She is particularly interested in child mental health, neurodevelopmental conditions, research ethics and qualitative methodology.

Dr. Ginny Russell is an interdisciplinary senior research fellow in mental health and developmental disorders at the University of Exeter Medical School in the UK. Her research interests encompass diagnosis, autism, ADHD and dyslexia. She has published over 40 journal articles and heads up a project using autism and neurodiversity to explore issues in diagnosis.

Dr. Steven J. Taylor is a historian of childhood and medicine. His research explores ideas and constructions of childhood health, lay and professional diagnoses, ability and disability, and institutional care. His first monograph, *Beyond the Asylum: Child Insanity in England, 1845–1907* was published by Palgrave Macmillan in 2017. He is currently researching the experience of special schools in the early twentieth century as a Wellcome Trust ISSF Fellow at the University of Leicester.

Dr. Jan Walmsley is an independent researcher and author specialising in the history of intellectual disabilities. She is a Trustee of Learning Disability England and a Trustee helper for self-advocacy group My Life My Choice. She is author of numerous books and papers. Her most recent book, edited with Simon Jarrett, is *Transnational Perspectives on Intellectual Disability in the Twentieth Century* (Policy Press, 2019). It brings together accounts of the recent history of intellectual disabilities in 12 countries across the world.

Dr. Imogen Wiltshire is an art historian and Wellcome Trust ISSF Postdoctoral Research Fellow at the University of Leicester. She specialises in modern and contemporary art, and her research focuses on the visual arts, health and medicine. She completed her Ph.D. in history of art at the University of Birmingham, funded by the Arts and Humanities Research Council (AHRC). She is currently writing a book on therapeutic art-making practices and modernism in Britain and the USA in the first half of the twentieth century. She is also working on a project about the artist Magdalena Abakanowicz.

List of Figures

List of Tables

CHAPTER 1

Introduction to Healthy Minds: Mental Health Practice and Perception in the Twentieth Century

Steven J. Taylor and Alice Brumby

Introduction

Writing in the 1980s, Peter Barham noted that 'in 1985 the average number of psychiatric beds occupied each day in England and Wales was 64,800, a return to the occupancy level last witnessed in 1895'.[1] In a local case study of the Exeter region, the number of inpatient beds in mental hospitals had fallen from 2070 in the middle of the twentieth century (1949) to only 100 beds in 1996. Ten years later, this number had dropped again to only 40 beds.[2] Similar figures can be found for different regions across the UK.[3] This reduction of provision in the country's mental hospitals and the narrative of deinstitutionalisation

S. J. Taylor (✉)
School of History, University of Leicester, Leicester, UK
e-mail: sjt48@leicester.ac.uk

A. Brumby
School of Humanities, Religion & Philosophy,
York St John University, York, UK
e-mail: A.Brumby2@hud.ac.uk

S. J. Taylor and A. Brumby (eds.), *Healthy Minds in the Twentieth Century*, Mental Health in Historical Perspective,
https://doi.org/10.1007/978-3-030-27275-3_1

communicates only a part of the history of mental health care over the course of the twentieth century.[4] While there was a sea change from institutional to social care in the provision and treatment of mental health, there was also a move beyond metaphorical walls that saw concerns about mental health penetrate previously untouched aspects of everyday life. The contributions to this book are an attempt at providing historical context to this change, as well as revealing some of the new physical and cultural spaces that mental health now occupies.

In economic, military, medical and social arenas, the twentieth century was one of change and development. As the century progressed, advances in surgery and medicine meant that people were living into older age, while, on the other hand, political and military situations demonstrated a prolificacy in destroying human life. The early decades of the century also saw a re-emphasis on the importance of the individual, their place in society and, alongside this, their health and well-being. Individuals were now tasked with an expectation of social efficiency that meant providing for themselves and their families but also, in their own way, contributing to the national project—whether through work, service or reproducing healthy stock. In this climate, minds considered to be 'unhealthy' were represented as a unique threat and took on a particular status that combined concern with stigma. From the degenerative worries of eugenic discourse through to the stresses and strains of modern living in the late-twentieth century, there was ever more awareness on preserving 'healthy' minds. Consequently, medical practices of removing the 'insane' from society and confining them in specialist institutions largely subsided and increased scientific, medical and sociocultural investment led to better understanding of conditions such as epilepsy, 'shell shock' and depression, as well as the emergence of new conditions such as schizophrenia, autism and post-traumatic stress disorder.

Throughout this volume, the terms 'healthy' and 'unhealthy' have no fixed meaning and are deployed subjectively in relation to the mental health of individuals and groups. The definitions have subsequently been determined by contributing authors in relation to a range of factors such as time, place and space. On the whole, the healthy/unhealthy dichotomy aims to identify instances where mental health was demarcated from what was considered socially, medically, culturally or legally 'normal'. Therefore, there is no single example of a healthy mind nor is there one of an unhealthy mind. To complicate the situation further, it might be that a mind might be considered unhealthy in some scenarios, and yet not in others. An example is that of learning disabilities; in Chapter 5, Jan Walmsley discusses some of the negative connotations and stigma attached to such conditions. Yet, in Chapter 8, authored by Dyck and Russell, the passage of time and changing cultural landscape of the twentieth century had shaped the experience of living with learning disability into something considered to be healthier, or socially accepted with the coming of the neurodiversity movement.

As the shifting understanding of what was considered to be a healthy mind suggests, and the chapters that follow will attest, the nomenclature of mental health was fluid and contested throughout the twentieth century. Thus, it is worth observing at the outset some of the terminologies that will feature. At the beginning of the twentieth century, the medical lexicon of mental health included terms such as 'lunatic', 'imbecile' and 'idiot' that all fell under the catch-all umbrella of 'insanity'. By the time that the century had ended, all of these medical terms had taken on derogatory connotations and were laced with stigma. The fate of these labels was not unique and the twentieth century saw language of its own—'feeble-minded', 'schiz' and 'cretin' related to mental health that fell into wider, negative, social use. As these terms feature in the academic analysis of this volume, it is worth observing that they are used by authors to demonstrate their arguments and with no malice or negativity in mind. Instead, terminology is used to reflect the historical nomenclature of the time period discussed.

The evolving language of mental health over the course of the twentieth century also reflects a widening social awareness of mental illness and disability. It was within this context that psychiatrists and medical experts became increasingly concerned with preventative mental health care, or the need to keep minds healthy. This fascination was the impetus behind a range of twentieth-century innovations, from charitable bodies to government policies, and societal doctrines. The preoccupation with maintaining and perpetuating healthy minds informed Eugenic discourse, the neo-hygienist child guidance movement, psychiatric social work and a host of legislation passed during the twentieth century—from the Mental Deficiency Act, 1913, to the policy of transition from treatment in mental hospitals to care in the community in the latter-half of the twentieth century. Nineteenth-century alienists, working in the field of mental health, often argued that late admittance to the asylum, and with it delayed treatment, led to the growing population of hopeless chronic cases, who languished in the institution uncured until their deaths.[5] In the twentieth century, there was a move away from cure, amelioration and modification, and the contributions to this volume from Dyck and Russell, Walmsley, and O'Reilly et al. reveal an advocacy and shared-identity towards mental health that would have been unimaginable a century before.

Places of Care for the 'Unhealthy' Mind

By the early to mid-twentieth century, overcrowding in asylums had highlighted, what appeared to be, the failure of institutionalisation. Subsequently, a range of other options emerged that attempted to ease pressure on over-crowded Victorian institutions.[6] To many, the late-nineteenth century symbolised a time of pessimism and decline in psychiatric services.[7] The argument that an increase in uncured chronic patients at the end of the nineteenth and early-twentieth centuries symbolised a period of stagnation within the walls of the asylum has been popularised by Andrew Scull.[8] Such a view has found traction in the literature, and Peter Bartlett stated that 'historians tend to view the asylum in the later-nineteenth century as a failure, full of incurable cases and unable to fulfil the humanitarian promise of the reformers'.[9] Echoing this perspective, Melling and Forsythe argued that the asylum model had 'exhausted its potential for innovation' long before 1890.[10] The growing demands upon care and the medical inability to cure the chronically ill are not disputed within this volume, nor is the idea that this growing 'underclass' of chronic patients can be seen, at some levels, to represent a failure in psychiatry at this time. Despite this, however, not all psychiatrists were negative and they saw ample reason for optimism in the range of new spaces for care in the twentieth century.[11] It is in these nascent spaces of treatment such as dedicated epilepsy services, special schools, sheltered employment, and patient and caregiver advocacy groups that contributions to this volume focus on.

Many of these newly emerging spaces were promoted and packaged as vehicles for reforming the field of psychiatry, which remained a contentious issue throughout the twentieth century. Critics writing in the second half of the twentieth century highlighted the regulatory nature of traditional asylums, branding them as being 'total institutions'.[12] Revisionist histories of asylum expansion in the late-nineteenth and early-twentieth centuries have tended to focus on issues of power and social control exerted by medical professionals over their patients.[13] These accounts modified older interpretations, which highlighted a humanitarian narrative focusing on psychiatry's progressive nature.[14] Critics argued that to focus solely on the humanitarian objectives of psychiatry was nothing more than an effort to legitimise and historicise the profession.[15] Arguably, creating new spaces of treatment and cure was an attempt not only to legitimise the psychiatric profession, but also to influence the (de)stigmatisation of mental illness across the long twentieth century.[16]

Despite the lingering images of mental institutions in the cultural imagination, historians have shown that the locus of care and treatment for those with mental health issues was never limited to the pauper lunatic asylum and, even in the nineteenth century, the economy of care sprawled across a range of settings in which the healthy and unhealthy mind could be presented, contested and represented.[17] These spaces and places included familial homes, boarding out with foster families, early mental health clinics, general hospitals and workhouse wards to name but the most popular.[18] Historians have come to accept that institutions were not closed, medicalised dumping grounds, but instead were porous, contingent and occasionally even temporary spaces where patients, staff, families and other stakeholders interacted.[19] Scholars have meticulously begun to show how the walls of the asylum were more permeable than our previous understanding suggests.[20] It is within the pluralistic landscape of care that this volume positions itself in an attempt to better understand the diverse physical and conceptual spaces that mental health came to penetrate in the twentieth century. In accordance with this broad and ambitious approach, the contributions to this volume span academic fields such as history, arts, literary studies, sociology and psychology, mirroring the diversity of the subject matter.

Healthy Minds, as a volume, contributes a new dimension to the study of mental health and psychiatry in the twentieth century. It takes the present literature beyond the 'asylum and after' paradigm to explore the multitude of spaces that have been permeated by concerns about mental well-being and illness. Unlike previous studies, the chapters in this volume consciously attempt to break down institutional walls and consider mental health through the lenses of institutions, policy, nomenclature, art, lived experience and popular culture. It also adopts a broad international scope covering the historical experiences of Britain, Ireland and North America.

Mental Health in the Twentieth Century: Policy and Practice

The Mental Deficiency Act, 1913, signalled a continuation of the nineteenth-century obsession with classifying and segregating individuals according to their mental health.[21] This legislation, dealing with so-called mental defectives, emphasised the dangers posed to society by those who previously might not have been the focus of medical experts. Subsequently, the new legal category of the 'feeble-minded' provided a label for individuals considered less severely disabled than 'idiots' and 'imbeciles', but 'weak-minded' enough to be more susceptible to crime, promiscuity and idleness.[22] Furthermore, the Act also established the Board of Control as a national body with overview of local authorities and their running of 'mental deficiency' services. Contributions to this volume by Jan Walmsley and Steve Taylor explore the impact of labelling and the consequences for individuals that this legislation targeted in more depth, both demonstrating the significance and lasting impact of its scope. Despite the eugenic appeal of this legislation, the pace of implementation was hampered by the First World War, restricted finances resulting from this conflict and the oncoming depression.

The Great War led to a crisis in the asylums of England and Wales as 27,778 permanent civilian beds were cleared and loaned to the Military Authorities to cater for injured personnel.[23] The result was devastating overcrowding in the remaining hospitals and a massive upsurge in asylum deaths.[24] Despite medical officers' best attempts, the 1920s continued to see an ever-increasing rise in the numbers of patients institutionalised.[25] It has been widely argued that the predominance of soldiers breaking down on the front led to some changes in the public view of mental illness.[26] However, the apparent inability of medical professionals to cure these men meant that any changes in attitudes were short-lived.[27] By the late 1920s, unrecovered 'shell-shocked' ex-servicemen found themselves languishing in asylums often alongside the chronically ill civilian population.[28]

By the time that the Mental Treatment Act, 1930, was passed, overcrowding in the nation's institutions for mental health had reached dire proportions.[29] Demand on services was so severe that hospital treatment was not always possible, and as such, patients often did not receive treatment until they reached an incurable stage of their illnesses.[30] The Mental Treatment Act, 1930, sought to prioritise early treatment by setting up categories of mental health care, which could bypass the lengthy certification process associated with previous experience. The act made provision for temporary and voluntary patients to be admitted to a mental hospital without the need for certification.[31] Importantly, it also championed the use of outpatient clinics and changed the name of the institution from an 'asylum' to a 'mental hospital' and reclassified 'pauper lunatics' to 'rate-aided' patients'. The change in nomenclature was clearly an attempt to remove the stigma from mental illness.[32]

Despite the hopes of the Mental Treatment Act, the Board of Control's desire to see mental health services reach parity with physical health did not occur properly until the founding of the National Health Service (NHS) in 1948. Even after services were officially aligned, mental health continued to remain the 'poor and embarrassing relative' of physical health in the popular imagination.[33] The Mental Health Act, 1959, attempted to alter this perception by repealing previous legislation relating to the Lunacy, Mental Treatment and Mental Deficiency Acts. By doing so, the distinction between psychiatric and other hospitals was fully removed.[34] However, the 1959 mental health legislation continued to justify compulsory detention for patients 'who may not know they are ill' and therefore may be unwilling to undergo treatment.[35] It was not until the Mental Health Act, 1983, where the ideas of consent were fully considered. Prior to this, in 1962, Enoch Powell produced his *Hospital Plan for England and Wales*, formally promoting the government's desire to dramatically reduce the number of inpatient mental hospital beds, and close down the hospitals by the end of the twentieth century. Of the 130 psychiatric hospitals in England and Wales in 1975, by 2005 only 14 remained open.[36]

Coinciding with a move towards non-institutional care in the 1960s was the emergence of the influential and popular anti-psychiatry movement.[37] In 1961, Thomas Szasz in his book *The Myth of Mental Illness* argued against the forcible detention of those who, he suggested, merely deviated from established societal norms.[38] Similarly, scholars such as Erving Goffman, Gilles Deleuze and Felix Guattari offered critiques of psychiatry's social influence and power and objected to the use of models and terms, inclusive of 'total institutions' that served to 'other' elements of the population.[39] Perhaps most famously, Michel Foucault in his seminal work *Histoire de la Folie* charted how attitudes towards the insane shifted with changing social values. He argued that psychiatry functioned as a tool of social control that began with a state-sponsored 'Great Confinement' of deviant populations.[40] Deinstitutionalisation evidently occurred at a time when arguments against psychiatry, and its social purpose, were gathering traction with more effective popular media vehicles.

Yet, while the closing of hospitals and focus on care in the community might sound unprecedented, it really was unique in size and scale alone. The move towards extramural forms of care was not exclusive to the mid-twentieth century, with outpatient departments available to those who did not require inpatient care pioneered as early as the 1890s.[41] Throughout this plotted history, we can see a desire to maintain the healthy mind, by classification and control, early treatment and the attempted removal of stigma, by endeavouring to bring mental health services in line with physical health. Whatever the legislation, there was an increasing focus on maintaining healthy minds and in doing so, maintaining a healthy society. If Bartlett and Wright's volume taught us that 'the boundaries between the asylum and the community are vague and uncertain',[42] then this volume identifies that throughout the twentieth century the boundaries between illness and wellness and the unhealthy and healthy mind can be similarly contested.

Keeping Minds Healthy: About the Chapters

Recent work has identified the importance of preventing mental illness and identifying its potential triggers, with Despo Kritsotaki et al. observing the modern nature of this particular focus.[43] In part, this volume seeks to answer the call for more research into this area, as the twentieth-century concentration on the healthy mind fits within this wider agenda of improved well-being and preventative mental health care. The objective of this book is to explore, what might be described as, the sprawl of mental health over the course of the twentieth century. This might be inelegant language, but there is a focus in the twenty-first century, at least in the Western world, on making sure that we are doing our best to keep our minds healthy. Cases in point are present-day concerns about the amount of time children, and adults, spend looking at digital screens; the negative effects of social media on everyday lives; anxieties about the body and self-image; and the consequences of substance abuse, particularly the emergence of synthetic drugs that are affordable and readily available. The contributions to this volume adopt an historical lens to help understand this present preoccupation with the healthy mind. Such an approach has meant that author contributions feature a diverse range of content, from traditional pauper lunatic asylums through to popular visual culture. Nevertheless, three broad themes, amongst others, emerge across the chapters that follow.

The first of these is the legal and medical classification of mental illness and disability, which has been a recurrent theme in the literature. At the beginning of the twentieth century, psychiatrists were fascinated with the distinction between mental health and learning disability, increasingly finding new ways of classifying those that they described as mentally defective and developing various gradations of the condition. The solutions that emerged to this supposed social problem were segregation of the afflicted, from society, as well as other populations of the insane, in order to create new physical spaces for their education and treatment.[44] Chapters by Steve Taylor and Jan Walmsley focus heavily on these emerging classifications and their significance. Walmsley, in particular, identifies the importance of labelling from a social perspective, while demonstrating the fluidity of language and the unintended legacies of medical classification.

With the publication of the *Diagnostic and Statistical Manual of Mental Disorders* (DSM) in 1968, and its subsequent iterations, psychiatrists were buoyed by an international classificatory system that was grounded in science and data. The contributions from Erika Dyck and Ginny Russell, Michelle O'Reilly et al. and Alice Brumby all explore how the new medical confidence in classification affected perception, stigma, treatment and lived experience of learning disability, autism and schizophrenia throughout the twentieth century. O'Reilly et al. discuss the evolution of autism, or as it has been described the 'twentieth-century disorder'. Their chapter highlights contested definitions, the challenges of applying labels to spectral disorders and the fractured nature of lived experience for those identifying as 'autistic'. Building on this, the chapter from Dyck and Russell examines how, in some circumstances, the identities created by medical classification fed into disability rights activism and the emergence of the Neurodiversity Movement (NDM) in the second half of the twentieth century. The growth of the NDM represented a complex relationship with medical labels, often appropriating medical languages such as 'patient', 'mad' and 'autistic' and redefining meanings to meet the specific needs of individuals at certain times and places. The nature of identity and experience is developed further in Alice Brumby's chapter. This contribution explores the growth of a relative's support organisation, which became the National Schizophrenia Fellowship, established in the 1970s. It aimed to meet the support needs of relatives and families by providing coping strategies that covered a variety of issues, ranging from stigma to caring for a family member. The use of oral history and archival material enables this chapter to argue that the friendship and support networks established by the Fellowship were an important way of dealing with the illness in the 'healthy minds' of non-schizophrenic relatives and caregivers.

The second theme that emerges is the plethora of places and spaces occupied by those living with unhealthy minds. These were mostly conceived by professionals or other stakeholders in a belief that they would be well-suited to treating or observing mental illness or disability. The volume opens with Alice Mauger's discussion of alcohol addiction in Ireland and the treatment of inebriates inside three institutions for lunatics. This chapter charts debates about alcohol-related lunacy and how it was best treated in a climate of nationalism and religion, and it particularly draws out the complicated relationship between alcoholism and the medical community's role in treating it. Moving outside of asylum walls, Rachel Hewitt considers diversifying institutional approaches to epilepsy treatment through an examination of specialist services in Britain and the USA between 1905 and 1965. She observes the similarities between epileptic colonies and open-air schools, marking a departure from asylum treatment and confinement for this class of patient. In these new spaces of well-being, walls were permeable, admission voluntary and treatment designed to improve the whole self. The colonies were about providing stigma-free employment and maintaining the healthy mind in spite of illness. This relationship between employment and the healthiness of the mind recurs in a number of chapters. Steve Taylor's chapter highlights how special education emerged at the beginning of the twentieth century as a mechanism for classifying and filtering those who could maintain independent lives from those that could not. In essence, state-sponsored education functioned as a measure of surveillance that sought to establish a healthy workforce while preventing the reproduction of unhealthy families. Moving later into the twentieth century, maintaining stigma-free employment in a safe space, despite an individual's disability, is central to the contribution from Andy Holroyde. Remploy was established in the UK in 1944 as part of the provision of the Disabled Persons Employment Act. It operated as a government-funded organisation that provided sheltered employment schemes for the disabled. Although it has been assumed that Remploy was originally for those of sound mind, Holroyde's chapter suggests that those with mental disabilities always had a role in the sheltered employment scheme. Allowing the mentally ill access to these services became increasingly important during the 1980s, to meet the need to provide care services, as an ever-increasing number of psychiatric institutions were closed down. Subsequently, sheltered employment became an important space in which healthy minds were promoted.

The final two chapters in the volume, from Imogen Wiltshire and Rob Mayo, link the theme of space with that of treatment. They focus on art, literature and film, as an important source of healing and well-being, and showcasing how the healthy mind has been represented and contested in the arts. Looking at a range of artistic and cultural practices, Wiltshire's contribution argues that these artistic movements were often at the centre of defining and creating healthy minds. The chapter identifies that in the first half of the twentieth century, the practice of viewing, making and creating art was associated with mental well-being. With a discussion that stretches from Surrealism to occupational and art therapy, the chapter illuminates a variety of historical relationships between art and mental health care. Moving into the world of popular science fiction in the latter half of the twentieth century, Rob Mayo's work focuses on inner space and dream-hacking as an important and influential sub-genre that focused upon the inner workings of the mind. The texts and films featured in Chapter 11 present popular twentieth-century understandings of how the mind works, the damage it can sustain and how it might be fixed. Many of the texts identify a hierarchy between the unhealthy mind and the healthy mind attempting to understand it. Echoing other chapters in the volume, the spaces that feature in the texts include a variety of locations, from the walls of a traditional abandoned asylum to non-institutional or non-psychiatric spaces.

Conclusions

Collectively the contributions to this volume look at a plurality of domains, spaces and places in which healthy and unhealthy minds have been represented, dissected and treated throughout the twentieth century. As the twenty-first century develops and a raft of new records becomes available, the twentieth century will become even more fruitful to historians. Perhaps the accessibility of sources has led to the dominance of studies into eighteenth- and nineteenth-century, predominantly institutional, mental health care. Historically, the rules on confidentiality and the destruction of records make twentieth-century records more difficult to access than nineteenth-century counterparts.[45] Despite this, however, research into twentieth-century institutions and loci of care are becoming more frequent within the historiography. Focusing on the twentieth century, and building on the work of Bartlett and Wright's influential edited collection *Outside the Walls of the Asylum*, this volume aims to look beyond the walls of psychiatric institutions. Certainly, throughout the twentieth century, health care professionals and policymakers have broadened and diversified the role of mental health care and opened up new spheres and centres for creating healthy minds. From the opening of child guidance and outpatient clinics to experiments with drugs, the twentieth century created new ways of policing and assessing the mind. This volume seeks to shed new light on these practices and centres which aimed to maintain the healthy minds of the collective and individual in a transnational context.

Notes

1. Peter Barham, *Closing the Asylum: The Mental Patient in Modern Society* (London: Penguin Books, 1992), 17.
2. A. Know and C. Gardner-Thorpe, *The Royal Devon and Exeter Hospital 1741–2006* (Exeter: Knox and Garner-Thorpe, 2008), 90–98.
3. Dylan Tomlinson, *Utopia, Community Care and the Retreat from the Asylums* (Buckingham: Open University Press, 1991), 42–66.
4. Nick Crossley, *Contesting Psychiatry: Social Movements in Mental Health* (London and New York: Routledge, 2006).
5. P. W. MacDonald, "Presidential Address on the Early Symptoms of Mental Disease and the Prevention of Insanity," *The British Medical Journal* 2 (October 1892): 885–887, 885.
6. Edward Hare, "Was Insanity on the Increase?" *British Journal of Psychiatry* 142, no. 1 (1983): 439–455; Andrew Scull, "Was Insanity Increasing? A Response to Edward Hare," *British Journal of Psychiatry* 144, no. 4 (1984): 432–436.
7. Sarah York, "Suicide, Lunacy and the Asylum in Nineteenth Century England" (Unpublished PhD thesis, The University of Birmingham, 2009), 35.
8. Andrew Scull, *The Most Solitary of Afflictions: Madness and Society in Britain, 1700–1900* (New Haven and London: Yale University Press, 1993), 271–272.

9. Peter Bartlett, "The Asylum and the Poor Law," in *Insanity, Institutions and Society: A Social History of Madness in Comparative Perspective*, eds. Joseph Melling and Bill Forsythe (London: Routledge, 1999), 48–67, 48.
10. Joseph Melling and Bill Forsythe, *The Politics of Madness: The State, Insanity and Society in England, 1845–1914* (London: Routledge, 2006), 6.
11. See Fredrick Lyman-Hills, "Psychiatry: Ancient, Medieval and Modern," *Popular Science Monthly* 60, no. 1 (1901): 31–48. See also Frank Crompton, "Needs and Desires in the Care of Pauper Lunatics: Admissions to Worcester Asylum, 1852–72," in *Mental Illness and Learning Disability Since 1850: Finding a Place for Mental Disorder in the United Kingdom*, eds. Pamela Dale and Joseph Melling (Oxon: Routledge, 2006), 46–64.
12. Michael Ignatieff, "Total Institutions and Working Classes: A Review Essay," *History Workshop Journal* 15, no. 1 (March 1983): 167–168.
13. Michel Foucault, *Madness and Civilisation: A History of Insanity in the Age of Reason* (London: Routledge, 1992); Erving Goffman, *Asylums: Essays on the Social Situation of Mental Patients and Other Inmates* (Harmondsworth: Penguin, 1986); Andrew Scull, *Museums of Madness* (London: Allen Lane, 1979).
14. Kathleen Jones, *A History of Mental Health Services* (London: Routledge and Keegan Paul, 1972); Richard Hunter and Ida Macalpine, *Psychiatry for the Poor: 1851 Colney Hatch Asylum—Friern Hospital 1973* (London: Dawsons Pall Mall, 1974).
15. Scull, *The Most Solitary of Afflictions*, 3.
16. Vicky Long, *Destigmatising Mental Illness? Professional Politics and Public Education in Britain, 1870–1970* (Manchester: Manchester University Press, 2014).
17. Peregrine Horden and Richard Smith, eds., *The Locus of Care: Families, Communities, Institutions and the Provision of Welfare Since Antiquity* (London: Routledge, 1998); Steven J. Taylor, *Child Insanity in England, 1845–1907* (Basingstoke: Palgrave Macmillan, 2017).
18. Peter Bartlett and David Wright, "Community Care and its Antecedents," in *Outside the Walls of the Asylum: The History of Care in the Community 1750–2000*, eds. Peter Bartlett and David Wright (London: The Athlone Press, 1999), 1–18.
19. Louise Wannell, "Patient's Relatives and Psychiatric Doctors: Letter Writing in the York Retreat, 1875–1910," *Social History of Medicine* 20, no. 2 (July 2007): 297–313; John K. Walton, "Casting Out and Bringing Back in Victorian England, Pauper Lunatics, 1840–70," in *The Anatomy of Madness: Essays in the History of Psychiatry*, eds. W. F. Bynum, R. Porter, and M. Shepherd (London: Tavistock, 1985), 132–146; David Wright, "Getting Out of the Asylum: Understanding the Confinement of

the Insane in the Nineteenth Century," *Social History of Medicine* 10, no. 1 (April 1997): 137-155; David Wright, *Mental Disability in Victorian England: The Earlswood Asylum, 1847–1901* (Oxford: Oxford University Press, 2001); Taylor, *Child Insanity in England*; Steven J. Taylor, "'She Was Frightened While Pregnant By a Monkey at the Zoo': Constructing the Mentally-Imperfect Child in Nineteenth-Century England," *Social History of Medicine* 30, no. 4 (November 2017): 748–766.

20. Graham Mooney and Jonathan Reinarz, eds., *Permeable Walls: Historical Perspectives on Hospital and Asylum Visiting* (New York: Rodopi, 2009). See also Bartlett and Wright, "Community Care and its Antecedents," 3.
21. Matthew Thomson, *The Problem of Mental Deficiency: Eugenics, Democracy and Social Policy in Britain, c.1870–1959* (Oxford: Oxford University Press, 2001). See also, David King, *In the Name of Liberalism: Illiberal Social Policy in the United States and Britain* (Oxford, Oxford University Press, 1999).
22. David Wright and Anne Digby, eds., *From Idiocy to Mental Deficiency: Historical Perspectives on People with Learning Disabilities* (London: Routledge, 1996); Mark Jackson, *The Borderland of Imbecility: Medicine, Society, and the Fabrication of the Feeble Mind in Late Victorian and Edwardian England* (Manchester: Manchester University Press, 2000).
23. Marriott Cooke and Hubert Bond, *History of the Asylum War Hospitals in England and Wales* (London: His Majesty's Stationary Office, 1920), 1.
24. John L. Crammer, "Extraordinary Deaths of Asylum Inpatients During the 1914–1918 War," *Medical History* 36, no. 4 (1992): 430–441.
25. For an illustration of the rise in numbers, see Scull, *The Most Solitary of Afflictions*, 369.
26. Elaine Showalter, *The Female Malady: Women, Madness and the English Culture, 1830–1980* (London: Virago Press, 1996); George Mosse, "Shell Shock as a Social Disease," *Journal of Contemporary History* 35, no. 1 (January 2000): 101–108, 101; Tracey Loughran, "A Crisis of Masculinity? Re-writing the History of Shell-Shock and Gender in First World War Britain," *History Compass* 11, no. 9 (2001): 727–738; Ben Shephard, *A War of Nerves: Soldiers and Psychiatrists in the Twentieth Century* (London: Pimlico, 2002).
27. Peter Barham, *Forgotten Lunatics of the Great War* (London: Yale University Press, 2007); Fiona Reid, *Broken Men: Shell Shock, Treatment and Recovery in Britain, 1914–1930* (London: Continuum, 2011).
28. Alice Brumby, "'A Painful and Disagreeable Position': Rediscovering Patient Narratives and Evaluating the Difference Between Policy and Experience for Institutionalised Veterans with Mental Disabilities, 1924–1931," *First World War Studies* 6, no. 1 (June 2015): 37–55.

29. West Yorkshire Archive Service (Henceforth WYAS), C85/1/6/10, Conference on Mental Hospital Accommodation (1931).
30. WYAS, C85/1/15/13, Annual Reports of the Board of Control (1929), 2.
31. The National Archives (Henceforth TNA), FD 1/1398, Copy of the Mental Treatment Act (1930).
32. Anon., "Mental Treatment: Improvements Under the New Act," *The Manchester Guardian*, 11 October 1930, 8. See also Alice Brumby, "From Pauper Lunatics to Rate Aided Patients: Removing the Stigma of Mental Health Care 1888–1938" (Unpublished PhD thesis, University of Huddersfield, 2015).
33. Mick Carpenter, "Forward: The Struggle Is Never Over," in *Mental Health Nursing: The Working Lives of Paid Carers in the Nineteenth and Twentieth Centuries*, eds. Anne Borsay and Pamela Dale (Manchester: Manchester University Press, 2015), xi.
34. Jed Boardman, "New Services for Old: An Overview of Mental Health Policy," in *Beyond the Water Towers: The Unfinished Revolution in Mental Health Services 1985–2005*, eds. Andy Bell and Peter Lindley (London: The Sainsbury Centre For Mental Health, 2005), 27–36.
35. Barham, *Closing the Asylum*, 131.
36. Lesly Warner, "Acute Care in Crisis," in *Beyond the Water Towers*, 38.
37. Nick Crossley, *Contesting Psychiatry: Social Movements in Mental Health* (London and New York: Routledge, 2006).
38. Thomas Szasz, *The Myth of Mental Illness: Foundations of a Theory of Personal Conduct* (New York: Harper & Row, 1961).
39. Erving Goffman, *Asylums: Essays on the Social Situation of Mental Patients and Other Inmates* (London: Aldine, 2007; originally published [New York: Anchor Books, 1961]); Gilles Deleuze and Felix Guattari, *Anti-Oedipus: Capitalism and Schizophrenia* (London: Athlone, 1984; first published *Capitalisme er Schizophrenie* [Paris: Les Editions de Minuit, 1972]).
40. Michel Foucault, *Madness and Civilisation: A History of Insanity in the Age of Reason* (London: Routledge, 2001; first published *Histoire de la Folie* [Paris: Plon, 1961]).
41. Anon., "Bethlem Royal Hospital by a Neurologist," *The Times*, 7 September 1888, 4; Louise Westwood, "A Quiet Revolution in Brighton: Dr. Helen Boyle's Pioneering Approach to Mental Health Care, 1899–1939," *Social History of Medicine* 14, no. 3 (2001): 439–457.
42. Bartlett and Wright, "Community Care," 12.
43. Despo Kritsotaki, Vicky Long, and Matthew Smith, eds., *Preventing Mental Illness: Past, Present and Future* (Basingstoke: Palgrave Macmillan, 2019).

44. See for instance, Thomson, *The Problem of Mental Deficiency*; Mark Jackson, *The Borderland of Imbecility*; Wright and Digby, *From Idiocy to Mental Deficiency*.
45. Westwood, "A Quiet Revolution in Brighton," 439–457.

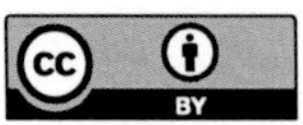

CHAPTER 2

'The Holy War Against Alcohol': Alcoholism, Medicine and Psychiatry in Ireland, c. 1890–1921

Alice Mauger

Introduction

In 1904, members of the Medico-Psychological Association (MPA) met at a conference in Dublin. On one point, attendees were practically unanimous, as evidence was produced 'from every side' of the 'disastrous effects everywhere observed' of drink. In response to this event, the *Journal of Mental Science* issued a rallying cry:

> It may cause some searching of conscience to ask whether our profession as a whole, and particularly our speciality, have up to the present taken a sufficient leading part in the holy war against alcohol. It is high time for our Irish colleagues to make themselves heard upon this subject, when in at least one asylum one third of the male admissions are attributed chiefly to this cause.[1]

A. Mauger (✉)
University College Dublin, Dublin, Ireland
e-mail: alice.mauger@ucd.ie

S. J. Taylor and A. Brumby (eds.), *Healthy Minds in the Twentieth Century*, Mental Health in Historical Perspective,
https://doi.org/10.1007/978-3-030-27275-3_2

Their shared sense of urgency—even culpability—is understandable. By now, Irish asylums had come to serve, among their catalogue of functions, as major receptacles for inebriates.[2] But this situation had never been deliberate. In spite of their outward preoccupation with the Irish 'drink problem', medical practitioners, late Victorian reformers and the state had reached little consensus on how best to deal with the chronically drunken. The short-lived system of inebriate reformatories, consigned to the shadows of criminality and the penal system, did little to tackle the professed 'epidemic' of inebriety sweeping through pre-Independence Ireland.[3] Meanwhile, members of the medical community contemplated alternatives ranging from treatment at home to physical force. While these practitioners continued to debate whether alcoholism was a cause of insanity—or insanity itself—by 1900, 'intemperance in drink' accounted for one in ten asylum admissions.[4] This chapter explores the evolution of medicine's role in framing and treating alcoholism in Ireland, from the 1890s until the creation of the Irish Free State in 1922.[5] Centring on medical discourses and asylum records, it queries how, why and to what extent medical practitioners came to influence the treatment, care and rehabilitation of alcohol-related admissions to Irish asylums.

This investigation marks a new departure in histories of alcohol use and misuse in Ireland. It also contributes to international discourses surrounding the role of medicine and particularly psychiatry, in understanding and treating alcoholism. Although Irish drink consumption patterns have been variously attributed to economic, legal, social and recreational changes, there has been little consideration of the rapidly professionalising medical community's attitudes towards excessive drinking and alcohol addiction at the turn of the twentieth century. Likewise, the long-held 'drunken Irish' stereotype, still prevalent, has been assessed from several viewpoints, but there has been no investigation of how the Irish medical community interpreted and informed this labelling. As this chapter demonstrates, Irish medical practitioners remained conscious of this racial typecasting. On the other side of the seemingly pervasive heavy drinking culture in Ireland, was the endurance of various temperance organisations boasting staggering membership figures.[6] Like their British colleagues, some Irish doctors were heavily influenced by temperance ideology. Meanwhile, as this chapter reveals, several asylum patients admitted for alcohol-related causes would take or had previously taken an abstinence pledge. The Irish relationship with alcohol was further complicated by the notion that sobriety was essential for successful national self-governance,[7] a position that was not lost on certain Irish doctors. As will be argued, while alcoholism was very much on the medical agenda internationally during this period, in Ireland it became imbued with a discrete set of cultural and political ideas.

Patient records for the Enniscorthy District Lunatic Asylum in the southeast of Ireland, the Belfast District Lunatic Asylum in the north of Ireland and St. Patrick's Hospital in Dublin are a key source in this study. Enniscorthy and Belfast were two of the twenty-two district (public) asylums which, by 1900, collectively housed almost 16,000 patients.[8] The state had authorised the creation of these institutions in 1817 for the 'lunatic poor', and they continued to serve that group almost exclusively.[9] St. Patrick's, meanwhile, was one of four voluntary asylums, all Dublin-based, which offered both private and non-private care. Founded from the bequest of Irish writer and dean of St. Patrick's Cathedral, Jonathan Swift in 1757, St. Patrick's initially received patients from all social classes but as the district asylums grew, fee-paying patients from the 'middling classes' increasingly came to form the patient population there. Importantly, there were also, by 1900, 13 private asylums, providing mostly expensive accommodation for the wealthiest members of society. Their role in caring for Ireland's inebriates is examined through official records, including the annual reports of the lunacy inspectors. From 1845, the inspectors—all medical men—were required to visit all 'receptacles for the insane' and reported annually on their observations. These doctors, who remained central figures in lunacy administration, also commented on the role Irish asylums played in treating alcohol-related disorders.

Medical Discourses

By the 1890s, there is little question that Irish medical practitioners, like their European and American colleagues, had come to redefine what we now term alcoholism as a disease rather than a vice.[10] Although the key features of the disease concept were in place by the 1770s, physicians including Thomas Trotter in Britain and Benjamin Rush in America have historically been credited as 'discovering' the disease view at the turn of the nineteenth century.[11] As Roy Porter has shown convincingly, this was because wider social developments at the dawn of the nineteenth century, including Evangelical Christianity, the temperance movement and the increasing status of medicine, were a crucial setting within which the disease concept could thrive.[12] It was at this point that doctors began outlining a specific medical condition. The term *Trunksucht*, literally meaning 'manic thirst', was coined in 1819 by the German-Russian doctor, C. von Brühl-Cramer, and was translated as 'dipsomania': a pre-existing condition giving rise to a craving for alcohol.[13] While for Brühl-Cramer, this was a disease of the *nervous system*, twenty years later, the renowned French alienist Jean Étienne Esquirol, contended that dipsomania was a *mental* disease, manifested by the inability to abstain from intoxicating liquor. Esquirol classified dipsomania as a form of partial insanity—monomania—a category he invented to diagnose patients who were unable to reason properly on one particular subject but were otherwise lucid.[14]

In the mid-nineteenth century, the Swedish doctor, Magnus Huss, provided the first clinical description of the disease he called 'chronic alcoholism'. By now, some form of disease theory had gained acceptance among many British doctors, including Alexander Peddie.[15] Yet while Peddie favoured Esquirol's conception of habitual drunkenness as a specific mental disease—dipsomania—Huss saw chronic alcoholism as a disease of the nervous system with a primarily physiological origin. These divisions were not clear-cut, however; in fact, the fluidity of medical thought in this era led to the terms often being used interchangeably. By the 1880s, another term—'inebriety'—had entered the fray, following its popularisation by the Glaswegian doctor, Norman Kerr. Inebriety differed in that it described an inability to resist all drugs rather than simply alcohol; meanwhile, Kerr tended to oscillate between 'alcoholism' and 'dipsomania' when discussing alcohol, while others often used 'inebriety' when referring solely to alcohol.[16] Kerr was the leading British champion of the disease (rather than 'vice') view. In 1884, he became a founding member and president of the British Society for the Study of Inebriety and soon after, published his *Inebriety, Its Aetiology, Pathology, Treatment and Jurisprudence* (1888), which became the standard text on the topic.[17]

In Ireland, the disease view gained currency in public arenas, as evidenced in the national and regional press.[18] Yet the belief, shared by many, that the drunkard was to blame for their condition and therefore deserved punishment was resilient.[19] As a review of Kerr's famous work *Inebriety* published in the *Dublin Journal of Medical Science* in 1888 illustrates concisely, this shift met with some resistance from Irish medical commentators. The review began:

> The main object of Dr Kerr's work seems to be to establish Inebriety (why not call it "Drunkenness"?) as a recognised disease, the prevention and treatmenttreatment of which comes within the province of medical men.

Although the reviewers subscribed to the importance of establishing a 'disease' framework, they criticised Kerr for seeming 'to neglect the moral responsibility of the intemperate, and their power of avoiding the exciting and continuing cause of the disease condition'.[20] As will be seen, while Irish doctors frequently looked to European and American examples when trying to solve Ireland's 'drink problem', they were not simply blind followers of international thought. Rather, they engaged with and informed wider international debates on inebriety, leaning on evidence gathered from practising medicine in Ireland. In the case of Kerr, now widely recognised as having been a leading specialist on inebriety,[21] the Irish medical community quickly warmed up. Just a year later, a review of the second edition of *Inebriety* in the same journal conceded that it had 'rapidly been adopted as a handbook', lauding the doctor's 'long and varied experience' and the 'illustrative and interesting cases' he presented.[22]

By the 1890s, Irish medical men, including Ephraim MacDowel Cosgrave, began publishing vigorously on inebriety and its treatment. Cosgrave, who trained in Ireland at Trinity College Dublin and qualified as a medical doctor in 1878, initially practised medicine in England. He later returned to Dublin, becoming a fellow (1887) and then president (1914–1916) of the Royal College of Physicians of Ireland, as well as physician to several Dublin hospitals.[23] Like Kerr, who was a member of the Church of England Temperance Society, Cosgrave was an enthusiastic temperance advocate and served as president of the Irish branch of the British Medical Temperance Association.[24] In 1897, he published a brief history of the Dublin Total Abstinence Society and in 1901, a book outlining experimental proofs on the role of alcohol.[25] In the meantime, he had become an active contributor to the *Dublin Journal of Medical Science*, which would later become the official organ of the Royal Academy of Medicine in Ireland.[26]

Cosgrave's views on inebriety were explicit in his presidential address to the Section of State Medicine at the Royal Academy of Medicine in Ireland in 1892 on 'the Control of Inebriates'. He advocated for extended powers for the treatment of inebriates and, perhaps predictably given his allegiance to temperance, recommended total abstinence as the only course for either class.[27] Sceptical of proposals that inebriates were best treated in their homes, he warned that due to their ingenuity, unscrupulousness and help from others, it would be difficult to keep them from drinking. Drawing on his personal experience as a hospital physician, Cosgrave determined that even in that environment, patients managed to acquire alcohol. He therefore urged the confinement of inebriates in institutions 'where they can be controlled – not allowed to have drink sent in, not allowed to go out for it'.[28] Like many of his contemporaries, Cosgrave was keenly aware of developments abroad citing legal developments in England, Scotland, America and Germany. For Cosgrave, inebriate homes, reshaped by new legislation, held the wonder-cure, though he insisted that power should be given to family, friends and public authorities to send people to them.[29] This marked a renewed campaign from the Irish medical community and the press for further institutional measures for chronic drunkards.[30]

It also mirrored developments in Britain. A key aim for Kerr's Society for the Study of Inebriety was to secure state-supported legislation which, it hoped, would establish medical treatment for inebriates and generate the expansion of the inebriate homes system. As Virginia Berridge has observed, the disease concept assumed hegemony in this period not due to the discovery of new medical ideas but because of a particular combination of social forces.[31] Thus, medical approaches to alcohol use were at least partly rooted in late Victorian ideological assumptions, as the disease model's entry into the public domain was not the achievement of a politically neutral scientific encounter but via the creation of quasi-penal institutions for the restraint and rehabilitation of the habitual drunkard.[32] For some historians, influenced by the ideas of Michel Foucault, these developments are evidence of the extension of the 'clinical gaze': the control of populations by pathologising and medicalising deviancy. Yet the lack of a unified disease theory of drunkenness, partly arising from the fact that inebriety sat uneasily with theories of rationality and reason, undermines this interpretation.[33]

Not all members of the Irish medical community were convinced of the need for further coercive legislation. In a particularly indignant backlash, the reviewers of the third edition of Kerr's *Inebriety* book wrote in the *Dublin Journal of Medical Science* in 1895:

> We object to the grandmotherly legislation and coercion. The liberty of the subject is sufficiently restricted already, and the patience with which millions of law-respecting citizens tolerate the curtailment of their personal liberty lest a weak brother should offend is a marvellous testimony to our inborn respect for law. Restrictions and pledges cannot create an Utopia.[34]

This tirade was almost certainly a reaction to the Intoxicating Liquors (Ireland) Bill and Irish Sunday Closing Bill, intended to introduce further restricted weekend opening hours for public houses. The reviewers' concerns resonated with contemporary nationalist sentiment at a time when Irish politicians were making strides towards Home Rule for Ireland.[35] In 1891, Charles Stewart Parnell, the then leader of the Irish Home Rule Party, had denounced the Intoxicating Liquors Bill as 'a patronising attempt on the part of the majority of English members in the House of Commons to make the Irish people sober'.[36] In fact, by this time, most Irish nationalists perceived 'attacks on Irish drinking habits as attacks on the Irish people', claiming that parliament was spending too much time on the drink question at the expense of more pressing concerns. The general consensus at this point was that the related issues of temperance and liquor licensing could be dealt with by an Irish legislature.[37]

While the reviewers of Kerr's book were not totally opposed to his arguments, they protested that he was a 'well-known advocate of teetotalism', 'pledges' and 'legal restriction against the consumption of alcohol'. They also condemned the author's use of his 'favourite illustration', the eradication of ether-drinking in County Tyrone, suggesting that it was the influence of Father Mathew's temperance campaign during the 1840s which had caused this problem in the first place:

> Thus from Cork to Belfast, Ireland is made a sober kingdom. But the peasant took neither to tea, coffee, nor Bovril. At fairs, wakes, and dances he found the so-called cordials, consisting of raw corn whisky and flavoured syrup in the south; and, in the thrifty north, methylated ether, was his panacea for trouble.[38]

Although they were pleased to observe the decline of ether consumption in the area by some 90%, a result of it being scheduled as a poison, the reviewers were anxious that alcohol should not follow suit and evoked the spectre of prohibition in the US state of Maine:

> Are we to christen publicans "druggists?" And are we, as in Maine, USA, to call on our pharmaceutical chemist for a "mint pick-me-up" instead of going to our hotel or public-house?[39]

The tirade did not end there. They concluded that:

> Reform never came from faddists. Their exaggerations disgust the unbiased. The work of making Great Britain and Ireland a sober nation is the work of the broad-minded common sense people in our midst.[40]

Alarm over the potential intrusion of further restrictive laws was slow to be realised, however. In fact, it was not until 1906, after twenty-eight years of debate, that a partial Sunday Closing Act was made permanent in Ireland.[41]

In spite of the Draconian spirit of some of Cosgrave's suggestions, the physician concluded by affirming his belief that:

> in many cases inebriety is a disease closely allied to insanity and susceptible of successful treatment, if power is given to keep the patient from drink for a sufficiently long period; and believing that the sooner the case is taken in hand the more is the probability of cure.[42]

There was nothing remarkably new about Cosgrave's alignment of inebriety with insanity. In fact, the belief that drunkenness caused madness had its roots in the late eighteenth century, where it was discussed in the works of physicians including Trotter and Rush. As we have seen, many influential alienists had adopted this framework and by the 1850s, it was widely accepted by medical men.[43]

Cosgrave's paper spawned mixed reactions. While the doctors present were unanimously courteous and expressed their gratitude to him for raising the topic, many offered contrasting solutions. Among them, one practitioner, a Dr. Davys, suggested that the only successful treatment or cure for the intermittent drinker was for a physician to recommend (with the family's approval) a strong male attendant who could be employed to 'wait on the inebriate, and by physical force prevent him taking any alcohol, the patient to be kept in the house'. According to Davys, this gave families much greater privacy and was bound to cure the drunkard within about three days. The same course should be adopted if (and often when) the 'patient breaks out again'. Apparently once patients returned to their sober state, they fully approved their treatment.[44]

The Medical Inspector of the Local Government Board, Edgar Flinn, diverged in his approach, urging that inebriates should be removed from the home and 'in some instances, they might with propriety be placed in asylums'.[45] This proposal was contentious and did not meet with agreement from most asylum doctors. Rather, as Mark Finnane has reasoned, the failure of inebriate reformatories and retreats gave rise to a scenario where the 'asylum was an easy last resort'.[46] In France, alienists were equally unsure about the suitability of asylums as treatment centres for alcoholics, who they blamed for the silting up of asylums, especially in Paris.[47] This issue gained increased attention in nineteenth-century Ireland, where the significance of alcoholism as a cause of insanity was contested.[48]

Alcoholism and Asylums

While the Irish psychiatric community had strong professional ties with its British counterpart, including several Irish members of the MPA[49] and Irish participation in the *Journal of Mental Science*, Irish asylum doctors did deviate from the frameworks of their British colleagues.[50] Coinciding with their appointment as lunacy inspectors in 1890, Drs. George Plunkett O'Farrell and E. Maziere Courtenay hastily warded off suggestions that asylums might offer care for those considered intemperate but not mentally ill.[51] But they were soon forced to recognise that voluntary patients no longer deemed insane but who wished to remain in private asylums hoping to recover from alcohol dependence could do so. Because voluntary boarders could neither be detained against their will, nor registered as lunatics, the inspectors concluded that their admission would benefit those unable to care for themselves at home.[52] By this time, some private asylums had clearly assumed the role of rehabilitation centres for those who could pay the high fees charged to lodge in them.

This is unsurprising, given that private asylum care was almost exclusively the preserve of the wealthy. Evaluating the feasibility of creating 'receptacles for dipsomaniacs' in 1875, the former lunacy inspectors, John Nugent and George William Hatchell,[53] speculated that drunkenness among the 'lower orders without social position or means' was treated as an offence or misdemeanour, while among the 'better and richer classes' it was often perceived as an 'incipient malady'.[54] For the rich, then, a tendency to overindulge in drink may have been viewed as more deserving of asylum care. In fact, during the late nineteenth century, private asylum patients were more likely to be admitted due to alcohol than the poorer patients sent to voluntary and especially district asylums. The reverse is true for Britain, where drink was less often identified as a symptom of illness among private asylum patients in England and was usually associated with the working classes in Scotland.[55]

If the lunacy inspectors were quite content for private asylums to function in this way, the ever-expanding state-funded district asylums were a different matter. In 1893, Courtenay and O'Farrell issued a circular to the resident medical superintendent (RMS) of each district asylum asking them to account for the alleged increase of insanity in Ireland. In response, they mostly concurred that insanity was not directly caused by alcohol.[56] This diverged from contemporary discourses in France and Britain where alcohol was cited as a chief cause.[57] In Ireland, some medical superintendents recognised excessive drinking as a manifestation of existing insanity, others cited adulterated alcohol as a cause, and still more believed that the habitual drunkard produced offspring liable to insanity, including epileptics.[58] These views had also been expressed by Cosgrave, who argued that the heredity fallout from inebriety caused neuroses in the descendants including hysteria, epilepsy and inebriety itself.[59] This was to be expected, given the well-established links between alcohol and degeneration which occupied much of the contemporary dialogue on the alleged increase of insanity in Ireland and elsewhere.[60] The rise of eugenics had influenced the campaign for Irish inebriate reformatories, where much of the attention was directed towards women's drinking.[61] Similarly in Britain, the major concern about alcohol was with the impact of women's drinking on the future of the race.[62]

While consensus had apparently been reached as to the hereditary nature of alcoholism, asylum doctors working in rural and urban districts made contrasting observations about the consequences of excessive drinking. In his response to the circular, L. T. Griffin, the RMS at the Killarney asylum, claimed:

> I cannot consider that with our rural population its abuse is a very prominent cause of insanity in this district. The peasant drinks to excess occasionally at fairs, weddings, wakes, & c., but he is not a habitual drinker, rather he is a total abstainer except on such occasions. However, this occasional debauch with its consequent poverty and insufficient food to the family, probably exercises an injurious influence, and so far the abuse of alcohol must be held to be a cause.[63]

By contrast, Edward D. O'Neill, the RMS at the Limerick asylum, wrote: 'there is not a shadow of a doubt abuse of alcohol swells our asylum population, not so much in country districts as in large towns and cities'.[64] In a similar vein, Conolly Norman, the renowned RMS of the Richmond asylum in Dublin (later known as Grangegorman), stated that in asylums which contained large urban populations, many cases were admitted directly due to drink while 'doubtless very many more' were indirectly related.[65] These responses support Catherine Cox's finding that while Irish asylum doctors' explanations for the alleged increase of insanity in Ireland were mostly in line with the British and European intellectual climate, they also drew upon their personal and cultural understandings of their patient populations.[66] Although those in the British countryside also tended to drink less than those in British towns and cities,[67] Ireland's overwhelmingly rural character posed a different paradigm for medical practitioners working in these areas.

The same can be said for the wider Irish medical community, for whom these arguments still resonated a decade later. In 1904, a reviewer of an issue of the British periodical, *The Medical Temperance Review* for the *Dublin Journal of Medical Science*, remarked:

> That a more than dimensional proportion of the interest of the alcohol question is justly due to Ireland is well known to its every intelligent inhabitant. The evils of alcoholism are spread out before our pain-stricken vision in every lane and alley of our metropolis; and, to a slighter degree, in all our towns and villages.[68]

The notion that sobriety was essential for successful national self-governance also coloured medical opinion. The reviewer went on to articulate the well-worn 'Ireland Sober, Ireland Free' dictum:

> One of the heaviest blows which a patriotic Ireland could possibly inflict on its neighbouring British rulers would be given by taking the pledge all round – old and young – and keeping it! Why, we often say to ourselves, do not patriotic politicians utilise this fact?[69]

This interpretation was by no means peculiar to Irish medicine. As Diarmaid Ferriter has shown, temperance campaigners were also alarmed by the recognition that the terms 'drink' and 'Irish' were becoming interchangeable in a caricature which was seen to diminish and downgrade Irish claims to independence.[70] Adherence to the well-known stereotype of the 'drunken Irish' was certainly visible among non-Irish contributors to the *Journal of Mental Science*. In 1900, an article described the year's 'statistics of drink' as 'puzzling' and appearing

> to prove some facts oddly at variance with common notions; for instance, that a luxurious use of intoxicating drinks is increasing in some circles in these islands, and that Englishmen are very much more drunken than Scottish or Irish folk.[71]

The Irish press seized upon statistics of this nature as evidence that they 'remove from our country the slur which British moralists would cast upon her'. Nonetheless, they were careful not to deny that 'intemperance is a terrible evil in our midst'.[72] Irish contributors to the *Journal of Mental Science*, however, did not respond to such findings, apparently choosing instead to remain largely silent on the issue. This perhaps reflected the distance many Irish asylum doctors perceived between themselves and their largely peasant patient population, pointing to class differences within the drink question more broadly, which were permeating psychiatry.

Calls for the Irish psychiatric community to engage in the 'holy war against alcohol' also reverberated with Irish temperance rhetoric. In 1899, Archbishop John Ireland had delivered a thundering address to the Irish Sunday Closing and Early Saturday Closing campaign in which he had incited a 'modern holy war' against excessive drinking and castigated the considerable number of public houses in Ireland.[73] At the 1904 MPA conference, the eminent RMS at the Enniscorthy District Lunatic Asylum, Thomas Drapes,[74] echoed the Archbishop, when he pointed out that 'there is one lunatic or idiot in Ireland to every 178 of the present population and one public-house to every 176!' Drapes observed that for the 'neurotic' and the person disposed to drink, every one of these ubiquitous public houses was an ever-recurring temptation.[75] While Drapes was especially resolute about the damaging effects of alcohol and showed keen support for temperance activities in his local community,[76] his views were also representative of a large segment of the Irish medical community. The doctor's apparent preoccupation with drink is predictable, given he, like many of his colleagues, was a protestant, Trinity-educated doctor of Anglo-Irish extraction. Following the demise of Fr Theobald Mathew's remarkably successful temperance 'crusade' in the 1840s, the temperance movement had come to be seen largely as the 'preserve of middle-class, pro-British protestants who used it to bolster their own position while at the same time denigrating the customs and habits of their Catholic social inferiors'.[77] Yet by the early twentieth century, some increasingly militant Irish nationalists were finding much in common with the new Catholic temperance movement, the Pioneers' Total Abstinence Association, particularly the renewed belief that sobriety held the key to Irish independence.[78] Thus, while Drapes was an unlikely ally of the nationalist cause,[79] some members of the Irish medical community were absorbing and even propagating their ideology. The heavily politicised nature of the Irish drink question in this era was clearly giving rise to multiple interpretations among doctors.

In spite of appeals to engage in the 'holy war', the Irish psychiatric community made little further remark on alcoholism in the ensuing decades. In 1912, two new lunacy inspectors, Drs. Thomas I. Considine and William R. Dawson, carried out a nationwide survey which examined the correlation between asylum committal rates and a range of social behaviours including alcohol consumption. Their findings led them to conclude there was no significant connection between asylum size and rates of drunkenness.[80] In their subsequent reports, they made no comment on the high rates assigned the cause of alcohol, although they continued to measure them. By this point, alcohol was coming to be viewed as a 'stumbling block' for the already 'unstable brain', again mirroring shifts in European contexts.[81] Discussion of the links between alcoholism and heredity also ground to a halt in the early twentieth century. In 1910, degeneration theory had become hotly contested when Karl Pearson and Ethel Elderton at the Galton Laboratory for National Eugenics at University College London found 'no discernible connection between parental alcoholism and mental defects in their children'.[82] Meanwhile, the 'increasing influence of the Freudian movement also hastened the end of degenerationist thought'.[83] The collapse of the inebriate homes system both in Ireland and in Britain also undermined medical authority, given the very public medical support for this initiative. As debates on the physiological and psychological effects of alcohol raged on in Britain throughout the First World War,[84] and in the United States, the seeds of prohibition were actively being sown, in Ireland, any further medical involvement in the drink question was apparently deferred until after the War of Independence (1919–1921) and subsequent partition (1922–1923) of the island into two separate states.

Diagnosing Alcoholism

In spite of the Irish psychiatric community's inertia in solving the drink question, in their daily practice asylum doctors regularly identified and attempted to treat alcohol-related illnesses. Asylum admissions related to alcohol remained consistently high in the decades leading up to independence. According to the lunacy inspectors, in 1890 one in eight men and one in twenty-two women were admitted to district asylums for 'intemperance'.[85] In December of that year, one in eleven men and one in twenty-six women were in voluntary and private asylums owing to 'intemperance in drink'.[86] In the last report published prior to independence in 1919, alcohol was considered the chief cause for one in sixteen patients and one of multiple factors for almost one in ten, with rates remaining higher for men than for women.[87]

While drink was very often identified as a *cause* of insanity, alcohol-related *diagnoses* were far less common. Among those admitted to district asylums in 1890, just one in seventeen men and one in thirty-five women were diagnosed with mania *a potu*, a form of insanity attributed to excessive alcohol consumption, which, like mania itself, was characterised by excited or violent symptoms and sometimes identified with delirium tremens.[88] Reflecting the approval of private asylums as suitable establishments for inebriates, mania *a potu* was more commonly diagnosed in patients admitted to voluntary and private asylums; in the same year, one in thirteen men and one in fourteen women were diagnosed with this disorder.[89] By 1909, the last year for which figures for mania *a potu* or any other alcohol-related disorder were included in the annual reports, this pattern was reversed with one in sixteen of men and one in fifty-six women sent to district asylums diagnosed with this disorder, compared to one in eighteen men and only one in 143 women sent to voluntary or private asylums.[90]

The trends are similar for patients admitted to Belfast, Enniscorthy and St. Patrick's asylums. Nearly all of the alcohol-related admissions to these institutions were attributed to alcohol. Of these 901 patients, 524 were assigned alcohol only, a further 246 were assigned the additional cause of heredity, but only 160 were diagnosed with an alcohol-related disorder. Instead, almost half were diagnosed simply with mania. This departs significantly from trends in the Sainte-Anne asylum in Paris, where diagnoses of alcoholism made up almost a quarter of male admissions, and was said to have contributed to a further 7.3%.[91] These divergences in diagnostic and aetiological categorisation in the Irish case reflect different medical understandings of alcoholism as a contributing factor of mental disorder rather than mental illness itself. Of course, the causes assigned tell us as much about lay, as they do medical definitions. The medical certificates which accompanied patients on admission allowed certifying doctors—usually not psychiatrists—to record cause of illness, and this was heavily based on information provided by family and friends. On admission, asylum doctors could then choose to confirm or alter this information.[92] While medical rather than lay authorities therefore had the final say over what was recorded, there is little doubt that the attitudes towards alcohol of those committing patients, including poor law and judicial official, friends, relatives and even the patients themselves, were represented.[93]

Case notes for individual patients shed light on the diverse criteria applied when citing alcohol as a cause of illness. Both the quantity of alcohol taken and the length of time a patient had been drinking varied widely. At Belfast, one patient assigned the cause of 'drink' had reportedly 'been drunk all his life', yet another had been drinking hard for only two weeks prior to taking ill, consuming '110 glasses of whiskey in the fortnight'.[94] Meanwhile, an Enniscorthy patient told his doctor that 'he occasionally drank a good deal of porter, up to 7 or 8 bottles in the day if he was out on duty or with friends but this would not incapacitate him from business'.[95] The criteria were equally eclectic at St. Patrick's. While Patrick D. was described as 'very intemperate – 1 pint at least of whiskey being taken for years daily', Patrick C. was said to have 'been drinking but not recently'.[96]

It is striking how frank many patients were in conversations with asylum doctors. This contradicts the general consensus among many Irish medical practitioners, discussed above, that the drunkard could not be trusted and usually denied their drinking. Patients and their relatives often attempted to rationalise why they drank to excess. As will be discussed later, the sheer number of public houses and resultant availability of drink was cited as a frequent cause for relapse among patients. Another common theme was the death of a loved one.[97] Maria D., admitted to St. Patrick's with 'alcoholic insanity' in 1904, was 'reported to have taken 1½ pints of brandy per day for some time'. She later stated that 'her intemperance was due to shock consequent upon the sudden death of her son'.[98] In a particularly heart-wrenching set of circumstances, Anne L. was admitted to Enniscorthy in 1904 for melancholia caused by the 'death of child and drink'. Anne had buried five or her six children who had all died under the age of eighteen months, and her husband stated that after the last child died, 'she fretted after him and he says people gave her whiskey. He can't say how much but too much'. Anne later confirmed her husband's explanation and was discharged recovered the same year.[99] Links between excessive drinking and mourning were not confined to female patients. When Patrick H. was admitted to Enniscorthy in 1909, diagnosed with acute melancholia, the causes assigned were 'predisposing: heredity; exciting: death of wife and children – drink'. Patrick presented himself at the asylum and asked to be taken in saying that his '"head was wrong" since the death of his wife and he feared he would do some harm to himself and thought of drowning himself in a hole of water'. Patrick's wife had died while giving birth to twins who both died nine days later.[100] Another patient, James J., told his doctor that 'ever since his father was drowned in the Noir [river] he has "been a fearful man for drinking"'.[101]

In a number of cases, both halves of a married couple reportedly drank to excess and were seen as a bad influence on one another.[102] The brother of one Enniscorthy patient told Drapes that 'he thinks it was his wife get him deranged, as she drinks too … he did a splendid business and was most popular, but thinks that it has gone more or less to [?] since both he and wife took to drink'.[103] Similarly, the brother-in-law of another patient, William McN, told Drapes he believed the patient's:

> Drinking and derangement were all due to his wife "who ought to be in the asylum instead of him". She drinks twice or thrice times what he'd drunk. Used to go away from him for 3 or 4 months and then when he had no comfort at home he would go to the publics [public houses] and drink mostly beer: little or no whiskey"… He says that he (patient) was convinced that his wife was trying to poison him. That he is a right good fellow and that every one of the neighbours "would die for him."

When William was discharged less than a month later and his wife came to collect him, Drapes noted that she had 'the aspect of a drinking woman'.[104] These examples correspond to Holly Dunbar's finding that women, and especially wives, were expected to steer men away from vices and towards sobriety.[105] Yet, at least in Enniscorthy, criticism of a patient's spouse was not limited to one gender. In 1906, patient Barbara B.'s illness was ascribed to both 'drink' and 'husband's intemperance' and the patient told Drapes that 'her attack was caused by annoyance of her husband drinking'. She did, however, admit to drinking up to 'two, four or even six bottles of porter' when they were given to her. On a visit from her husband, the assistant medical officer, Dr. Hugh Kennedy, clearly sympathised with the patient, writing of her husband that 'he had drink taken and attempted to beat her – when prevented by Attendant Hanna Fenlon became very cheeky and abusive'.[106] Cases like these demonstrate that in the eyes of medical staff, both husbands and wives were potentially corrupting influences on their spouses.

Insight into the type of people admitted to asylums for excessive drinking or alcoholism can also be gleaned from patient records. A typical case for the period from 1890 to 1921 was a man in his thirties or forties, who had usually been married, was Roman Catholic and had worked in either the agricultural or industrial sector. The much higher level of male admissions is expected, given that alcoholism has historically been viewed as a male problem.[107] Thus, while men were often over-represented, especially among those committed to rural asylums,[108] they were considerably more likely than women to be described as suffering from alcohol-related illnesses (between 67.7 and 87%). Prestwich has found similar in her study of alcoholics committed to the Sainte-Anne asylum in Paris, reflecting the lack of public medical attention geared towards female alcoholism in the late nineteenth and early twentieth centuries.[109] By the First World War, however, there was well-documented alarm over female alcoholism, in both Ireland and abroad. Dunbar has chronicled the contemporary revulsion for women who drank excessively during the First World War in Ireland, a theme which Prestwich has identified in the French context.[110] These anxieties have been linked to women's changing role in society, while alcoholism in women was often associated with sexual immorality.[111] Notably, women's excessive drinking may have more frequently been seen as criminal, as they were more likely to be sent to inebriate reformatories than men.[112]

The occupational profile of male patients in this study contrasts somewhat with Prestwich's characterisation of male alcoholic patients admitted to the Sainte-Anne asylum in Paris, who 'with the exception of those in the wine and alcohol trades, were more likely to be vagabonds and unskilled or skilled workers and less likely to be drawn from the petty bourgeois categories of clerks and shopkeepers'.[113] Predictably, the 'agricultural class'[114] made up three-fifths of rural Enniscorthy's male alcohol-related admissions. The 'industrial class', which includes dealers, publicans, shoemakers, carpenters, shopkeepers and tailors, was well represented in both Enniscorthy (21%) and Belfast (36.8%), while the professional and commercial classes were over-represented among patients sent to Belfast (12.8%) and St Patrick's (14.3%). In fact, those in the 'indefinite and non-productive class' are a good deal lower than the national picture.[115] While this may tell us more about the recording process than implying higher levels of employment among alcohol-related admissions, the figure of 40% unemployment among (male and female) alcohol-related admissions to St. Patrick's is at odds with Malcolm's finding that by 1884, nearly two-thirds of the general patient population had no occupation.[116] What is clear is that the men committed to the asylums studied were by no means unproductive layabouts, who had long ceased to provide for themselves and their relatives. To use the dictum of the time, they might be considered those who had fallen on hard times or the 'deserving poor'.

The same can be said for the female patients, who were over-represented in the industrial classes at both Belfast (27.6%) and Enniscorthy (19.1%) compared to the national figure of 8.1% in 1911. This group included weavers, dressmakers, spinners, dealers and mill-workers. In international contexts, occupations like 'dressmaker' have been revealed as euphemisms for prostitute and some known prostitutes in Ireland were returned in the 1901 census as dressmakers, housekeepers, waitresses and milliners.[117] However, given that the occupations of seven patients (3.8%) in this study were explicitly recorded as prostitute, it is unlikely that this was the case here. The proportion of women recorded as having 'no occupation' is also low by the standards of total district asylum populations, for whom this was usually the largest category, followed by those in the agricultural class.[118] This high level of employment mirrors that of women admitted for alcoholism to the Sainte-Anne asylum, who were also disproportionately likely to have worked outside the home. In the Parisian context, women in certain occupations, including cooks, laundresses and male and female wine traders, were reported to have regularly 'drank on the job'.[119] Again, this could be seen as reflecting anxieties about increased activity of women in the workplace and by extension, in the public sphere.[120] This line of thought has been visible in modern discourses, where since the 1980s the growing visibility of women in the workforce has given rise to the stereotype that women performing 'men's work' have come to replicate 'men's vices'. Conversely, and as Prestwich has argued, given their knowledge that working-class women led 'hard lives', French psychiatrists accepted that women, like men, might develop job-related or occupational alcoholism.[121]

Another defining characteristic of alcohol-related admissions to asylums was the short periods of time they tended to remain incarcerated.[122] Like most asylum patients, half the patients in this study stayed for less than six months. Longer stays of five years or more accounted for only 17.6% compared to over a quarter of all asylum patients.[123] Those admitted to St. Patrick's stayed the shortest length of time, with almost three quarters released within the first year. Gender apparently impacted on rates of discharge: women were slightly less likely (58.2%) than men (66.5%) to be released within a year while they were more likely (15.3%) than men (10.1%) to become long-term patients of ten years or more. Those who stayed longer had much higher chances of dying in the asylum, with 71.1% of those staying between five and ten years and 93.2% of those staying ten years or more doing so. Short-term patients, on the other hand, had very high chances of recovery: 73.1% of those released within six months were described as 'recovered' and a further 12.3% as 'relieved'. Repeated admission, a substantial characteristic in all Irish asylums, was also a remarkably strong trait among those suffering from alcohol-related illness, both in Ireland and internationally.[124] While tracing readmissions is not an exact science, at the very least, one in ten patients in this study was returned to the asylum and references to previous confinements in other institutions were not infrequent. Unlike those readmitted to the Sainte-Anne asylum, who after two or three times were deemed incurable, readmissions did not seem to impact negatively on the outcome of patients' stays.[125] In fact, many of those admitted repeatedly were likely to be discharged recovered.

Treating Alcoholism

The high level of readmissions speaks volumes about the lack of effective treatment and implies that the general lack of medical consensus about alcoholism and mental illness translated to asylum practice. Similar to the regime at the Ennis State Inebriate Reformatory,[126] treatment for alcoholic excess or addiction largely followed the ordinary asylum regime of good feeding, fresh air and exercise, and occupational therapy.[127] Given the overcrowding in most district asylums, there were less recreational facilities for patients at Belfast and Enniscorthy. Life in a voluntary asylum like St. Patrick's was apparently more varied, and patients were occupied at games like billiards and draughts, playing the piano, cycling and going for drives.[128] There were a number of commercial cures on the market both internationally and in Ireland, especially at the turn of the century, ranging from hypnotism to Dr. Keeley's infamous 'gold cure' (injections of bichloride of gold) to the 'Normyl' cure for Alcohol and Drug Addictions (twenty-four days of a medicine which was 75% strychnine).[129] Yet, aside from the use of strychnine in Enniscorthy and St. Patrick's asylum, such cures were apparently not administered.[130] Likewise, several of the treatments employed at German, Swiss and French clinics, including the traditional hydrotherapy and massage, and more experimental gymnastics and sunbathing, did not gain currency in Ireland.[131]

In contrast to the State Inebriate Reformatory, where there was very little recourse to drug therapy or specific cures, in Irish asylums a number of drugs, particularly sedatives, were given to patients, usually soon after admission when the effects of drink were at their height.[132] These included hyoscine, mophia, digitalis, paraldehyde, trional, potassium bromide and sulphonal. When other treatments failed, solitary confinement was used in some exceptional and usually violent cases. After John George F., a patient admitted to St. Patrick's asylum 'became violently delirious' he was put into a padded room 'in a typical state of delirium tremens'. When he was deemed to be 'out of his deliriums', he was released after a total confinement of fifty-nine hours and ten minutes.[133] Similarly in 1906, Enniscorthy patient Andrew S. was put in a padded room and given 1/96 grains of hyoscine.[134] The need to manage violent patients did not apparently extend to mechanical restraint, however. When Thomas R. was brought in from the New Ross Workhouse in a straightjacket in 1909, Kennedy insisted it be 'removed at once'.[135]

Abstinence was another important tenet of treating alcoholic excess or addiction and naturally one which patients found the most difficult to endure. Several patients requested alcohol while in the asylum. At St. Patrick's, Cecelia Frances W. told her doctor 'she would appreciate some good wine', while William G. R. complained of not being given '"Chablis & Chianti" wine … Frequently asks the writer [asylum doctor] for a drink out of the bottle of Port Wine which he says he sees in my pocket'.[136] At the Ennis Reformatory, the minimum period of detention and therefore abstinence was eighteen months but as we have seen asylum patients were frequently released within a few months.[137] Moreover, and in spite of the British and Irish medical communities' increased hostility towards drink and reluctance to prescribe it as medicine, several patients were given drink in the asylums studied.[138] Surprisingly, it was the keen temperance activist, Drapes who most often recorded giving his patients drink. In 1891, he wrote 'I tried substituting bot[tle] of porter for 2 oz of wine but tho' he said he would like it, he can with difficulty be got to take even some of it'.[139] Five years later, he gave another patient some 'whiskey as she was deadly pale and her pulse very weak'.[140] This reflects the duality in medical attitudes towards alcohol in this era, wherein many doctors retained their faith in the therapeutic and restorative qualities of alcohol, while acknowledging the dangers of alcohol abuse.[141]

Although more than half the patients in this study whose outcome is known were discharged 'recovered' and a further 11.7% 'relieved', the long-term effects of asylum treatment were clearly not succeeding in many cases. The lack of aftercare options in Ireland posed profound challenges for those released from asylums. While Germany boasted a 'network of support groups to assist former drinkers', there were no such organisations in Ireland, save for a handful of philanthropic and state-funded societies for discharged prisoners.[142] Prestwich has noted that in the absence of post-cure care in France, the re-education of the drinker was continued by families, support groups and abstinence organisations.[143] Similarly in Ireland, the only forms of support outside the asylum were apparently families and the temperance movement, and patients were actively encouraged to take the pledge upon release. In fact, a condition of release for several Enniscorthy patients was their promise to do so.[144] Yet, a number of patients were evidently unable to remain abstinent. In 1902, James J., who had been admitted to Enniscorthy previously with mania *a potu* said he kept the pledge for two years, but had started drinking again in the two weeks leading up to his committal. He was again discharged recovered after less than one month in the asylum, and Kennedy later noted: 'keeping very well lately. He took the pledge on Saturday and if he keeps it should be all right'. However, about two weeks later he provided the following update: 'heard he is just as bad as ever and drinking again'.[145] In the same year, William W. also diagnosed with mania *a potu* 'said he had the pledge till lately, when he began to drink again; whiskey and porter and everything he could get: that he had been at work steadily up till then'. On discharge it was stated, 'he appears quite well in mind and has taken the Pledge'.[146] In some cases, patients actually cited the pledge as the root of their mental distress. John K., who was admitted to Enniscorthy with alcoholic insanity, said 'he drank freely up to a month ago when he took the pledge. That he has been feeling depressed since then, esp. about something he did wrong at confession'.[147] At other times, patients were coerced into taking the pledge. In 1908, Enniscorthy patient Peter C. spoke of how he was forced by his brother, a priest, to do so.[148] This complicates our understanding of those who took the pledge in rural Ireland, especially the idea that Irish attitudes towards drinking were polarised between those who abstained and those who drank excessively.[149]

As we have seen, the Irish medical community was well aware of the temptation to drink in Irish society, not least because of the ready availability of alcohol in the abundant public houses. The father of one Enniscorthy patient, Philip F., told the assistant medical officer, Kennedy that he had asked 'the Publicans in Kiltealy not to give him drink. When they refused to supply him, he used to walk about three miles to get it'.[150] According to Dr. Oscar Woods, the RMS of the Cork asylum in 1894, 'in a large number of cases people who have just come out of the asylum are greeted with, "Oh! I am so glad to see you home; come and have a drink" and this is too often repeated, and a relapse brought on'.[151] Woods' interpretation was proven accurate time and time again among patients in this study. When Thomas McG was discharged from the Belfast asylum in 1914:

> He immediately went to a Public House and became intoxicated, he then went home to his father's house and threatened them. His father had him removed to the Union Infirmary and owing to his violent behaviour there he was re-certified.

He later escaped from the asylum:

> Assisted by some unknown friend who came for him in a Taxicab and bringing a suit of clothing. He went home to his father's house where he spent the night, leaving in the early morning to travel to Lisburn, Lurgan and Portadown. Unable to obtain work, he returned to Belfast and enlisted. Then becoming under [the] influence of alcohol returned to his father's house and during a quarrel with his father attempted suicide. He was arrested by the police and after being charged was transferred to the [Belfast Union Infirmary] and ultimately was brought back to the District Asylum at 10.30pm.

The same patient was discharged and readmitted to the asylum twice more before eventually being discharged recovered in 1917.[152] Other patients managed to abstain for slightly longer periods of time. Richard C. L., a solicitor who was discharged from St. Patrick's in 1911, 'resumed his former habits within ten days and as a result lost his appointment'.[153] The following year, W. J. McM, a bank clerk:

> On being discharged he, prior to taking up duties in a new office in Londonderry, went to Queenstown for a week & resumed his drinking habits there. On taking up his duties in Londonderry he gave up the drinking & after a few days became nervous and obsessed with a fear that he would make mistakes in money etc. & felt his memory going & so he returned at once.[154]

As Finnane has correctly contended, a publican's occupation was perceived as a specifically constant source of temptation.[155] In 1894, Catherine G., a barmaid in her sister's public house admitted to drinking porter while she worked there. As soon as she came into the asylum, she asked Drapes for a bottle of porter which he did not give her.[156] In 1914, Peter C., a publican diagnosed with mania *a potu* had suffered several attacks of delirium tremens at home. He was readmitted to Enniscorthy in 1914 having left only a week previously. According to the case notes, he started to drink as soon as he got out: 'He is drunk at present and staggering gait. Before leaving here he promised to go to a sister in the country for a few weeks but he went to his shop and began drinking'. He was discharged a few months later but less than a month after that was brought back 'blind drunk on admission', a pattern which continued several more times. There is no record of his eventual outcome.[157]

This cycle of relapse and recovery proved highly frustrating for asylum doctors, who, like their European colleagues, questioned the suitability of asylums as treatment centres for alcoholics.[158] By 1904, Drapes had become so exasperated by the repeated readmission of habitual drunkards to Enniscorthy that he blamed excessive drunkenness in Wexford for an increase of insanity there.[159] Drapes, however, appeared less frustrated than his predecessor, Joseph Edmundson, who had written of one patient: 'An habitual drunkard whom in my opinion a month on the treadmill in gaol would have a more permanent effect on than a month under kind asylum treatment'.[160] Edmundson was not alone in his rather harsh assessment. Some French doctors also recommended incarceration over asylum treatment, while one argued that 'amateur alcoholics' treated the asylums as a 'holiday retreat' in periods of seasonal unemployment.[161] Asylum care was clearly the preferable option for some patients. In 1909, Charles Henry B., who had previously been in prison wrote to his friend from St. Patrick's 'I never had a better time in my life getting as fat as a bullock which you will see'.[162] Even those who had not served penal sentences, like Mary C., a 50-year-old widow sent to Enniscorthy, appeared to almost enjoy their period of confinement. When Mary was discharged, it was noted that she 'had got to like the place and cried at leaving. Said she would rather stay longer with us'. She was readmitted soon afterwards.[163] By 1914, Drapes was replicating Edmundson's sentiments, when, following the discharge of Peter C., he received a letter from the patient's wife informing him 'Peter is just as bad as ever again. He started the drink as soon as he got home'. In response, Drapes recommended that 'if he got at all violent to have him arrested and sent to prison, which might have a more deterrent effect on him in future than a stay at the asylum. Otherwise told her she could send him back here'. As we have seen, the following year he was readmitted to the asylum 'blind drunk on admission'.[164]

Kennedy also grew increasingly weary. When Thomas C was brought to the asylum by the police, for having 'attempted suicide by hanging when in the cell at Police Station', Kennedy remarked scornfully:

> This is his old game, he always "attempts" suicide when arrested for being drunk and gets sent in here instead of being sent to jail. He replied quite readily and rationally to all questions and appears just as well as when he left here. He has "a screw lose" but is not really insane and knows well what he is doing.

Two months later, although the patient was showing progress and working at painting seats for the asylum, Kennedy reasserted his belief that he 'should have been sent to Jail not here'.[165] Kennedy was also resigned to repeated alcohol-related admissions. On the occasion of Thomas MacD's seventh discharge from Enniscorthy in 1908, Kennedy wrote 'as soon as he gets out he will start drinking again and be sent back here'. Kennedy was proven right when Thomas was again readmitted less than five months later.[166]

Aside from their lack of ability to permanently 'cure' alcoholism, and the professional embarrassment this must have entailed, a key issue for district asylum doctors was most likely the additional strain these patients were putting on the already overcrowded asylum system.[167] Notably, doctors at voluntary and private asylums demonstrated greater compassion towards alcohol-related cases. In 1920, the proprietor of the Lindeville private asylum in Cork, Dr. J. Osborne, wrote to the assistant medical officer at St. Patrick's Hospital's, Dr. H. R. C. Rutherford following the transfer of a former patient to St. Patrick's. In this letter, which was written to provide a case history for the patient, Osborne concluded 'I hope for his sake that he has recovered as he is quite a nice fellow. I should be very grateful if you would let me know in a week or two as I am most interested'.[168] There is also evidence of asylum doctors keeping in touch with former patients. For example, Arthur Q., a patient who had been admitted to St. Patrick's with alcoholic insanity, wrote to the hospital's medical superintendent, Dr. Leeper in 1906 following his discharge:

> Mr Dear Dr Leeper
> Very many thanks for your kind letter it was good of you to write so soon. I am so glad you got good sport in Wicklow I only wish I had been with you ... I must again thank you for all the kindness you showed to me and hope soon again to see you.
> Very sincerely yours, Arthur Q[-].[169]

Of course, with a much smaller patient population to manage, it is likely that the pressure on those working in private and voluntary asylums was less.

Conclusions

The sustained influx of alcohol-related admissions to Irish asylums sparked debate among the medical and psychiatric communities about the exact nature of alcohol addiction and how best to treat it. In line with wider European medical thought, for much of the two decades following 1890, most identified alcohol abuse as part of a greater trend towards degeneration. It is important to note, however, that Irish asylum doctors did not indiscriminately follow the commentary of their international colleagues. Guided by the differing social, cultural and political contexts of practising medicine in Ireland, including the enduring caricature of the Irish as a 'drunken' race and associations between the nationalist cause and the concept of healthy minds (in this case sobriety), they were quick to identify regional, cultural and class differences among their own patient populations. The taking of the abstinence pledge by many of the patients examined points to the influence of religion among the largely Roman Catholic populations in rural Irish asylums. In a largely rural country, where alcoholism was apparently more widely recognised as an illness among the rich and a vice among the poor, wealthier individuals were more likely to receive treatment in an asylum, while even those committed to the state-funded district asylums tended to be drawn from the 'respectable poor'.

Despite increased recognition of alcoholism as a disease in the decades before Irish independence and in an era when medicine was rapidly professionalising, the Irish medical community's role in treating alcoholism was apparently a reluctant one. This reflects the uncertainty shared by many asylum doctors as to the precise relationship between alcohol and insanity, the difficulties inherent in attempting to treat alcoholic cases and bearing in mind the seemingly relentless expansion of the district asylum system into the twentieth century. While this evident reluctance allows us to dismiss Foucauldian notions of the clinical gaze being extended towards alcoholism, it is likely that the rising influence of medicine and psychiatry in this era was, at least partially, responsible for the pathologising of alcoholism both in Ireland and internationally.[170]

Acknowledgements I would like to thank the Wellcome Trust for kindly supporting the research that this chapter is based on. Grant ref. 205455/Z/16/Z.

Notes

1. Anonymous, "Intemperance," *Journal of Mental Science* 50, no. 208 (January 1904): 117–118.
2. Mark Finnane, *Insanity and the Insane in Post-Famine Ireland* (London: Croom Helm, 1981), 146–150.
3. Calls for inebriate reformatories in Ireland were eventually met in 1898. The Inebriates Act of that year extended to Ireland and allowed for the committal of criminal inebriates to state or charitable-funded reformatories if they were tried and convicted of drunkenness at least four times in one year. But what medical reformers (both in Britain and in Ireland) had been campaigning for, that is, the compulsory power to detain non-criminal inebriates, never became law. In Ireland, the 1898 Act led to the establishment of four institutions.

But of these four, only the Lodge Retreat in Belfast accepted voluntary inmates and these were limited to fee-paying, protestant women. The remaining three institutions could only be accessed by those committed through the courts. These were the State Inebriate Reformatory in Ennis, and St. Patrick's and St. Brigid's certified inebriate reformatories for Roman Catholic men and women, respectively. This system was short-lived and, like Britain, had all but disappeared by the end of the First World War. See Conor Reidy, *Criminal Irish Drunkards: The Inebriate Reformatory System 1900–1920* (Dublin: The History Press Ireland, 2014); Elizabeth Malcolm, "Between Habitual Drunkards and Alcoholics: Inebriate Women and Reformatories in Ireland, 1899–1919," in *Gender and Medicine in Ireland 1700–1950*, eds. Margaret H. Preston and Margaret Ó hÓgartaigh (New York: Syracuse Press, 2012).

4. Finnane, *Insanity and the Insane*, 146.
5. Following the signing of the Anglo-Irish Treaty of December 1921, which ended the Irish War of Independence, Ireland was partitioned into two states. The twenty-six southern counties were reconstituted as the Irish Free State, an independent dominion of the British Commonwealth. The remaining six counties in the northeast of Ireland were formed into the state of Northern Ireland. This political partition of Ireland remains in place today.
6. See, for example, Diarmaid Ferriter, *A Nation of Extremes: The Pioneers in Twentieth-Century Ireland* (Dublin: Irish Academic Press, 1999); Elizabeth Malcolm, *'Ireland Sober, Ireland Free': Drink and Temperance in Nineteenth-Century Ireland* (New York: Syracuse University Press, 1986).
7. Ferriter, *Nation of Extremes*; Diarmaid Ferriter, "Drink and Society in Twentieth-Century Ireland," *Proceedings of the Royal Irish Academy* 115C (April 2015); Malcolm, *Ireland Sober, Ireland Free*.
8. *Fiftieth Report of the Inspectors of Lunatics (Ireland)* [CD 760], H.C. 1901, xxviii, 487.
9. Finnane, *Insanity and the Insane*, 18–52.
10. For an overview of medical understandings of alcoholism in international contexts, see Virginia Berridge, *Demons: Our Changing Attitudes to Alcohol, Tobacco & Drugs* (Oxford: Oxford University Press, 2013).
11. Berridge, *Demons*, 66–67; Roy Porter, "The Drinking Man's Disease: The 'Pre-history' of Alcoholism in Georgian Britain," *British Journal of Addiction* 80 (1985): 385–396.
12. Porter, "The Drinking Man's Disease."
13. Berridge, *Demons*, 88; James Nicholls, *The Politics of Alcohol: A History of the Drink Question in England* (Manchester: Manchester University Press, 2009), 66–67; F. W. Kielhorn, "The History of Alcoholism:

Brühl-Cramer's Concepts and Observations," *Addiction* 91, no. 1 (January 1996): 121–128.

14. Peter McCandless, "'Curses of Civilisation': Insanity and Drunkenness in Victorian Britain," *British Journal of Addiction* 79 (1984): 53.
15. Ibid.
16. Nicholls, *Politics of Alcohol*, 167–168.
17. Virginia Berridge, "The Origins and Early Years of the Society 1884–1899," *British Journal of Addiction* 85 (1990): 991–1003.
18. For example, "Drunkenness a Disease—Hospitals for Inebriates," *Kerry Weekly Reporter*, 28 June 1890, 6; "The Treatment of Drunkards," *Freemans Journal*, 7 December 1893, 4.
19. Finnane, *Insanity and the Insane*, 171n41; Malcolm, "Between Habitual Drunkards and Alcoholics," 119. For the British context, see McCandless, "Curses of Civilisation."
20. Review of Norman Kerr, "Inebriety: Its Etiology, Pathology, Treatment, and Jurisprudence," *Dublin Journal of Medical Science* LXXXVI (July–December 1888): 41.
21. Berridge, *Demons*, 90; Mariana Valverde, "'Slavery from Within': The Invention of Alcoholism and the Question of Free Will," *Social History* 22, no. 3 (1997): 255.
22. Review of Norman Kerr, "Inebriety," *Dublin Journal of Medical Science*, 314–315.
23. C. J. Woods, "Cosgrave, Ephraim MacDowel," in *Dictionary of Irish Biography*, eds. James McGuire and James Quinn (Cambridge: Cambridge University Press, 2009), 13.
24. Woods, "Cosgrave, Ephraim MacDowel," 13; "British Medical Temperance Association," *Freemans Journal* (23 June 1898), 13.
25. Ephraim MacDowel Cosgrave, *Brief History of the Society* (Dublin: Corrigan & Wilson, 1897); Ephraim MacDowel Cosgrave, *Experimental Proofs of the Role of Alcohol* (London: Ideal Publishing Union, 1901).
26. From 1874 to 1919, the *Dublin Journal of Medical Science* was edited by John William Moore; Thomas Gillman Moorhead was appointed co-editor in 1907.
27. Ephraim MacDowel Cosgrave, "The Control of Inebriates," *Dublin Journal of Medical Science* XCIII (January–June 1892): 179–180. For more on the concept of drunkenness as a disease of the will in international commentary, see Valverde, "Slavery from Within."
28. Cosgrave, "Control of Inebriates," 181.
29. Ibid., 183. Cosgrave also discussed the possibility of introducing a register for drunkenness based on a model currently used in Prince Edward's Island. See ibid., 185.

30. Malcolm, "Between Habitual Drunkards and Alcoholics," 111.
31. Berridge, "The Origins and Early Years of the Society."
32. Nicholls, *Politics of Alcohol*, 162.
33. See Berridge, *Demons*, 69; Nicholls, *Politics of Alcohol*, 168–169; Mariana Valverde, *Diseases of the Will: Alcohol and the Dilemmas of Freedom* (Cambridge: Cambridge University Press, 1998), 49.
34. Review of Norman Kerr, *Inebriety: Its Etiology, Pathology, Treatment, and Jurisprudence* (3rd edition), *Dublin Journal of Medical Science* XCIX (January–June 1895): 50.
35. Under the Act of Union in 1801, the Kingdom of Ireland was dissolved and Ireland was incorporated into the UK of Great Britain and Ireland. Beginning in the 1870s, a campaign began among Irish representatives in Westminster to secure a devolved government for Ireland. This was termed 'Home Rule'.
36. Cited in Malcolm, *Ireland Sober, Ireland Free*, 271. See also, Elizabeth Malcolm, "Temperance and Irish Nationalism," in *Ireland Under the Union: Varieties of Tension (Essays in Honour of T. W. Moody)*, eds. F. S. L. Lyons and R. A. J. Hawkins (Oxford: Clarendon Press, 1980), 94–98.
37. Malcolm, "Temperance and Irish Nationalism," 93–95.
38. Review of Norman Kerr, "Inebriety," *Dublin Journal of Medical Science* (3rd edition), 49.
39. Ibid.
40. Ibid., 50.
41. Malcolm, *Ireland Sober, Ireland Free*, 273–274.
42. Cosgrave, "Control of Inebriates," 185.
43. McCandless, "Curses of Civilisation," 49. See also W. F. Bynum, "Chronic Alcoholism in the First Half of the Nineteenth Century," *Bulletin of the History of Medicine* 42 (1968): 160–185.
44. "Section of State Medicine," *Dublin Journal of Medical Science* XCIII (January–June 1892): 327–328.
45. Ibid. Edgar Flinn was educated at Clongowes and the Royal College of Surgeons in Ireland and served twenty-five years in the Volunteer and Territorial Forces, retiring with the rank of Colonel. From 1895 to 1910, he was Medical Inspector of the Local Government Board in Ireland, and he was then appointed medical member of the Irish Prisons Board and Chief Inspector of Reformatories and Industrial Schools. See "Col. D. Edgar Flinn—Former Medical Inspector of Prisons, Dead," *Irish Independent*, 20 August 1926, 4.
46. Finnane, *Insanity and the Insane*, 147–148.

47. See, for example, Patricia E. Prestwich, "Drinkers, Drunkards and Degenerates: The Alcoholic Population of a Parisian Asylum, 1867–1914," *Histoire Sociale/Social History* 27, no. 54 (1994): 321–335.
48. Catherine Cox, *Negotiating Insanity in the Southeast of Ireland, 1820–1900* (Manchester: Manchester University Press, 2012), 60.
49. David Healy, "Irish Psychiatry, Part 2: Use of the Medico-Psychological Association by its Irish Members—Plus ça Change!" in *150 Years of British Psychiatry*, eds. Hugh Freeman and German E. Berrios (London: Athlone Press, 1996), 314–320.
50. For more on the place of Irish psychiatry within the British psychiatric community, see Fiachra Byrne, "Madness and Mental Illness in Ireland: Discourses, People and Practices, 1900 to c. 1960" (PhD diss., University College Dublin, 2011). This paragraph features research from Alice Mauger, *The Cost of Insanity in Nineteenth-Century Ireland: Public, Voluntary and Private Asylum Care* (Basingstoke: Palgrave Macmillan, 2018), 153, 154, 155–156.
51. *Fortieth Report of the Inspectors of Lunatics (Ireland)* [C. 6503], H.C. 1890–1891, xxxvi, 521, 189–90.
52. *Forty-Seventh Report of the Inspectors of Lunatics (Ireland)* [C. 8969], H.C. 1898, xliii, 491, 33.
53. O'Farrell and Courtenay succeeded John Nugent (1847–1890) and George William Hatchell (1857–1889).
54. *Twenty-Forth Report on the District, Criminal, and Private Lunatic Asylums in Ireland*, H.C. 1875 [319] xxxiii, 18.
55. Lorraine Walsh, "A Class Apart? Admissions to the Dundee Royal Lunatic Asylum, 1890–1910," in *Sex and Seclusion, Class and Custody: Perspectives on Gender and Class in the History of British and Irish Psychiatry*, eds. Jonathan Andrews and Anne Digby (Amsterdam and New York: Rodopi, 2004), 262; Charlotte MacKenzie, *Psychiatry for the Rich: A History of the Private Madhouse at Ticehurst in Sussex, 1792–1917* (London: Routledge, 1992), 152. See also McCandless, "Curses of Civilisation," 52.
56. *Forty-Third Report of the Inspectors of Lunatics (Ireland)* [C. 7466], H.C. 1894, xliii, 401, 187; Cox, *Negotiating Insanity*, 60, 62.
57. Prestwich, "Drinkers, Drunkards and Degenerates," 325; McCandless, "Curses of Civilisation," 50.
58. *Forty-Third Report of the Inspectors of Lunatics (Ireland)*, H.C. 1894, 187; Cox, *Negotiating* Insanity, 60, 62.
59. "Section of State Medicine," 328. For Britain see McCandless, "Curses of Civilisation," 55.
60. Cox, *Negotiating Insanity*, 61.
61. Malcolm, "Between Habitual Drunkards and Alcoholics," 111.

62. Berridge, *Demons*, 89.
63. *Forty-Third Report of the Inspectors of Lunatics (Ireland)*, H.C. 1894, 206.
64. Ibid., 214.
65. Ibid., 222.
66. Catherine Cox, "Managing Insanity in Nineteenth-Century Ireland" (PhD diss., University College Dublin, 2003), 65. See also Brendan Kelly, *Hearing Voices: The History of Psychiatry in Ireland* (Newbridge: Irish Academic Press, 2016), 96–100.
67. Berridge, *Demons*, 32; McCandless, "Curses of Civilisation," 52.
68. "The Medical Temperance Review," *Dublin Journal of Medical Science* CXVIII (July–December 1904): 139.
69. Ibid., 140.
70. Ferriter, *Nation of Extremes*, 5.
71. "The Strife with Alcohol," *Journal of Mental Science* 46, no. 194 (July 1900): 526.
72. "Untitled," *Evening Herald*, 6 April 1901, 4.
73. Ferriter, *Nation of Extremes*, 26.
74. Drapes published energetically on insanity and became the editor of the *Journal of Mental Science* in 1912. For more on Drapes, see Kelly, *Hearing Voices*, 93–96.
75. "Intemperance," 117.
76. Kelly, *Hearing Voices*, 93–96.
77. Malcolm, "Temperance and Irish Nationalism," 113. See also, Malcolm, *Ireland Sober, Ireland Free.*
78. Malcolm, "Temperance and Irish Nationalism," 111–115; Ferriter, *Nation of Extremes.*
79. In 1894, Drapes had cited the 'hopes, fears and anxieties' caused by constant political agitation, combined with the 'eloquence' of 'political teachers', as factors in the alleged increase of insanity in Ireland. Thomas Drapes, "On the Alleged Increase of Insanity in Ireland," *Journal of Mental Science* 40 (1894): 532. Also cited in Cox, *Negotiating Insanity*, 53–65. Additional evidence for this can be inferred from the fact there was no mention of nationalist activity in Drapes' obituaries. For example: "Thomas Drapes," *Journal of Mental Science* 66, no. 273 (April 1920): 83–87; "Dr Thomas Drapes," *Irish Times*, 7 October 1919, 4.
80. Cox, *Negotiating* Insanity, 62.
81. Ibid., 61–62. Daniel Pick, *Faces of Degeneracy: A European Disorder, c.1848–c.1918* (Cambridge: Cambridge University Press, 1989), 201–202.
82. Berridge, *Demons*, 91.

83. Ibid., 92.
84. Nicholls, *Politics of Alcohol*, 176.
85. *Fortieth Report of the Inspectors of Lunatics (Ireland)*, H.C. 1890–1891, 47.
86. Ibid., 88.
87. *Sixty-Seventh Annual Report of the Inspectors of Lunatics (Ireland)* [CMD 32], H.C. 1919, xxv, 305, ix.
88. *Fortieth Report of the Inspectors of Lunatics (Ireland)*, H.C. 1890–1, 48.
89. Ibid., 89.
90. *Fifty-Eighth Report of the Inspectors of Lunatics (Ireland)* [CD 4760], H.C. 1909, xxxii, 32, 17, 59.
91. Prestwich, "Drinkers, Drunkards and Degenerates," 325.
92. Cox, *Negotiating Insanity*, 220.
93. McCandless, "Curses of Civilisation," 50.
94. HOS/28/1/14/1/1 Belfast District Lunatic Asylum Casebook: Males, c. 1900–1926, George G; HOS/28/1/14/1/2 Belfast District Lunatic Asylum Casebook: Males, c. 1900–1935, William A.
95. Enniscorthy District Lunatic Asylum Clinical Record No. 3, 1891–1892, Bernard C.
96. St. Patrick's Hospital E/137 Casebook: Males, Patrick T; St. Patrick's Hospital E/137 Casebook: Males, Patrick C.
97. Prestwich has also noted this cause in the French context see Patricia E. Prestwich, "Female Alcoholism in Paris, 1870–1920: The Response of Psychiatrists and of Families," *History of Psychiatry* 14, no. 3 (2003): 328.
98. St. Patrick's Hospital E/141 Casebook: Females, Maria B.
99. Enniscorthy District Lunatic Asylum Clinical Record No. 9, 1903–1904, Anne L.
100. Enniscorthy District Lunatic Asylum Clinical Record No. 14, 1909, Patrick H.
101. Enniscorthy District Lunatic Asylum Clinical Record No. 3, 1891–1892, James J.
102. Prestwich has also noted the 'corrupting influences of others' as a cause in the French context see Prestwich, "Female Alcoholism in Paris," 328.
103. Enniscorthy District Lunatic Asylum Clinical Record No. 4, 1893–1894, Michael S.
104. Enniscorthy District Lunatic Asylum Clinical Record No. 5, 1895–1896, William McN.
105. Holly Dunbar, "Women and Alcohol During the First World War in Ireland," *Women History Review* (2016): 4.
106. Enniscorthy District Lunatic Asylum Clinical Record No. 12, 1906–1907, Barbara B.
107. For example, Prestwich, "Female Alcoholism in Paris," 321–22, 325; Cox, *Negotiating Insanity*, 222.

108. Elizabeth Malcolm, "'The House of Strident Shadows': The Asylum, the Family and Emigration in Post-Famine Rural Ireland," in *Medicine, Disease and the State in Ireland, 1650–1940*, eds. Elizabeth Malcolm and Greta Jones (Cork: Cork University Press, 1999), 178–179; Finnane, *Insanity and the* Insane, 131; Cox, *Negotiating Insanity*, 138.
109. Prestwich, "Drinkers, Drunkards and Degenerates"; Prestwich, "Female Alcoholism in Paris."
110. Dunbar, "Women and Alcohol During the First World War"; Prestwich, "Female Alcoholism in Paris," 322.
111. Berridge, *Demons*, 93–94; Dunbar, "Women and Alcohol During the First World War in Ireland."
112. Malcolm, "Between Habitual Drunkards and Alcoholics."
113. Prestwich, "Drinkers, Drunkards and Degenerates," 325.
114. Discussion of occupation profile in this chapter uses the classification system adopted in the General Report on the Census of Ireland, 1911. See *Census of Ireland, 1911. General Report, with Tables and Appendix* [CD 6663], H.C. 1912–1913, cxviii.
115. *Census of Ireland, 1911.*
116. Elizabeth Malcolm, *Swift's Hospital: A History of St Patrick's Hospital, Dublin, 1746–1989* (Dublin: Gill and Macmillan, 1989), 204.
117. Maria Luddy, *Prostitution and Irish Society 1860–1940* (Cambridge: Cambridge University Press, 2007), 45.
118. Malcolm, "House of Strident Shadows," 180.
119. Prestwich, "Female Alcoholism in Paris," 329.
120. Berridge, *Demons*, 93–94; Dunbar, "Women and Alcohol During the First World War."
121. Prestwich, "Female Alcoholism in Paris," 322, 329.
122. This is rendered more pronounced, given the declining discharge rates and increasing duration of treatment in some asylums after 1900. See Cox, *Negotiating Insanity*, 144. Prestwich has found similar for male patients at the Sainte-Anne asylum in Paris. See Prestwich, "Drinkers, Drunkards and Degenerates," 327.
123. Malcolm, "House of Strident Shadows," 180.
124. Ibid., 180–181. Prestwich, "Drinkers, Drunkards and Degenerates," 329.
125. Prestwich, "Female Alcoholism in Paris," 327.
126. Malcolm, "Between Habitual Drunkards and Alcoholics," 113; Reidy, *Criminal Irish Drunkards*, 41–62.
127. For more on treatment regimes in district asylums, see Finnane, *Insanity and the Insane*, 190–208; Cox, *Negotiating Insanity*, 207–230.
128. For example, St. Patrick's Hospital E/137 Casebook: Males, Benjamin Lloyd R.; St. Patrick's Hospital E/142 Casebook: Males, Robert T. For

more on the disparities in recreational activities between public and voluntary/private institutions in Ireland see Mauger, *The Cost of Insanity*, 196–201.

129. See Berridge, *Demons*, 73; Valverde, "Slavery from Within," 252. For Ireland, see, for example, "Hypnotism," *Freemans Journal*, 13 April 1891, 5; *Kerry Sentinel*, 21 November 1894, 4; "A Keeley Institute for Ireland," *Skibbereen Eagle*, 23 January 1897, 2.
130. For example, Enniscorthy District Lunatic Asylum Clinical Record No. 12, 1906–1907, Thomas O'B.; St. Patrick's Hospital E/145 Kalamazoo Casebook: Males, Richard C. L.
131. Patricia E. Prestwich, "Paul-Maurice Legrain (1860–1939)," *Addiction* 92, no. 10 (1997): 1261.
132. Reidy, *Criminal Irish Drunkards*, 59; Malcolm, "Between Habitual Drunkards and Alcoholics," 113.
133. St. Patrick's Hospital E/142 Casebook: Males, John George F.
134. Enniscorthy District Lunatic Asylum Clinical Record No. 12, 1906–1907, Andrew S.
135. Enniscorthy District Lunatic Asylum Clinical Record No. 14, 1909, Thomas R.
136. St. Patrick's Hospital E/141 Casebook: Females, Cecelia Frances W.; St. Patrick's Hospital E/142 Casebook: Males, William G. R.
137. Reidy, *Criminal Irish Drunkards*, 58.
138. Brian Harrison, *Drink and the Victorians: The Temperance Question in England, 1815–72* (London: Faber, 1971), 298–347; Malcolm, *Ireland Sober, Ireland Free*, 326.
139. Enniscorthy District Lunatic Asylum Clinical Record No. 3, 1891–1892, Philip D.
140. Enniscorthy District Lunatic Asylum Clinical Record No. 5, 1895–1896, Winifred K.
141. McCandless, "Curses of Civilisation," 51.
142. Prestwich, "Paul-Maurice Legrain," 1260; Reidy, *Criminal Irish Drunkards*, 64–65.
143. Prestwich, "Paul-Maurice Legrain," 1260.
144. For example, Enniscorthy District Lunatic Asylum Clinical Record No. 3, 1891–1892, Thomas M.
145. Enniscorthy District Lunatic Asylum Clinical Record No. 8, 1901–1902, James J.
146. Ibid., William W.
147. Enniscorthy District Lunatic Asylum Clinical Record No. 6, 1897–1898, John K.
148. Enniscorthy District Lunatic Asylum Clinical Record No. 13, 1908, Peter C.

149. For more, see Ferriter's study of the Irish temperance organisation, the Pioneers Total Abstinence Association: Ferriter, *Nation of Extremes.*
150. Enniscorthy District Lunatic Asylum Clinical Record No. 7, 1899–1900, Richard K.
151. Cited in Daniel Hack Tuke, "Increase of Insanity in Ireland," *Journal of Mental Science* 40, no. 171 (October 1894): 559.
152. HOS/28/1/14/1/4 Belfast District Lunatic Asylum Casebook: Males, c. 1916–1935, Thomas McG.
153. St. Patrick's Hospital E/145 Kalamazoo Casebook: Males, Richard C. L.
154. Ibid., W. J. McM.
155. Finnane, *Insanity and the Insane*, 150.
156. Enniscorthy District Lunatic Asylum Clinical Record No. 4, 1893–1894, Catherine G.
157. Enniscorthy District Lunatic Asylum Casebook 1 Clinical Notes, Admissions from 1909 to 1929, Peter C.
158. See Prestwich, "Female Alcoholism in Paris"; Prestwich, "Drinkers, Drunkards and Degenerates"; Cox, *Negotiating Insanity*, 61.
159. Finnane, *Insanity and the Insane*, 147.
160. Enniscorthy District Lunatic Asylum Clinical Record No. 4, 1893–1894, Bartholomew C.
161. Prestwich, "Drinkers, Drunkards and Degenerates," 329–330; Prestwich, "Female Alcoholism in Paris," 327.
162. Letter attached to St. Patrick's Hospital E/145 Kalamazoo Casebook: Males, Charles Henry B.
163. Enniscorthy District Lunatic Asylum Clinical Record No. 5, 1895–1896, Mary C.
164. Enniscorthy District Lunatic Asylum Casebook 1 Clinical Notes, Admissions from 1909 to 1929, Peter C.
165. Enniscorthy District Lunatic Asylum Clinical Record No. 9, 1903–1904, Thomas C.
166. Enniscorthy District Lunatic Asylum Clinical Record No. 13, 1908, Thomas MacD.
167. As already noted, French asylum doctors shared these concerns. See Prestwich, "Drinkers, Drunkards and Degenerates."
168. Letter appended to St. Patrick's Hospital E/145 Kalamazoo Casebook: Males, James B. M.
169. Letter appended to St. Patrick's Hospital E/142 Casebook: Males, Arthur Q.
170. See Berridge, *Demons*, 69; Nicholls, *Politics of Alcohol*, 168–169; Valverde, *Diseases of the Will*, 49.

CHAPTER 3

Social Stigma, Stress and Enforced Transition in Specialist Epilepsy Services 1905–1965

Rachel Hewitt

Introduction

For many people with epilepsy, the central characteristic of their impairment is fear. From a belief in supernatural possession to a ban on types of employment, people with epilepsy have historically faced stigma associated with the fear of seizures.[1] As Penny Rhodes et al. have argued, epilepsy sits in an awkward position within disability studies and indeed within the history of mental health.[2] The 'impairment' of epilepsy is often one that is invisible. Many people with epilepsy are thus often able to 'mask' their impairment, only being 'unmasked' after experiencing a seizure.[3] For this reason, according to Rhodes et al., people with epilepsy occupy an awkward position within the disability studies movement. Barriers to employment, access to services and the maintenance of social relationships are and have historically been shaped by the stigma surrounding seizures, which in itself creates a unique concept

R. Hewitt (✉)
Centre for the Social History of Health and Healthcare, Glasgow, UK
e-mail: Rachel.Hewitt@gcu.ac.uk

S. J. Taylor and A. Brumby (eds.), *Healthy Minds in the Twentieth Century*, Mental Health in Historical Perspective,
https://doi.org/10.1007/978-3-030-27275-3_3

of 'impairment', one not unlike that experienced by people with mental illness. The history of epilepsy has therefore largely been unwritten. Temkin's assertion that the history is a triumph of 'science over superstition' relates largely to the development of neurology as a science and omits people's experiences of specialist services, in spite of these services' domination in constructing the scientific knowledge of epilepsy. This chapter reflects the complex interplay between a variety of nascent twentieth-century scientific discourses, including psychiatry, psychology, and social policy, and their influence on people's experience of epilepsy.

G. Berrios argued that at the end of the nineteenth century, epilepsy was seen as separate from insanity.[4] Yet, people with epilepsy at the end of the nineteenth century were almost indistinguishable from those with hysteria and manic schizophrenia.[5] Localisation by John Hughlings Jackson in the 1870s, in addition to Jean Charcot's work in Paris, had created an explicit medical link between seizures and emotional and psychological states.[6] In particular, post-seizure states of automatism, confusion and irritability had led to a development of the idea that epilepsy was a psychological as well as neurological phenomenon.[7] The nineteenth century was the springboard for research into the medical causes of epilepsy—the twentieth century, however, saw a diversification of epilepsy research and services into the issues surrounding stigma, access to medication, childhood experiences and the importance of well-being. The site of the majority of this research was specialist services, developed from the 1870s. This chapter draws on sources of three epileptic 'colonies' in the UK and one 'colony' in Sonyea, NY, in the United States. The British colonies focused on in this chapter are now major UK charities representing people with epilepsy—the David Lewis Centre, Young Epilepsy, Epilepsy Action and the Epilepsy Society. Records for these colonies are scarce and, where they have survived, give an incomplete picture of the true experiences of young people within the colonies. In part, this reflects the chaotic nature of service transition and the complex map of service provision for people with epilepsy in the twentieth century. Extensive record-keeping allows for a more complete picture of life within the colony at Sonyea; however, there is limited data on transition, reflecting widely different approaches to institutionalisation and deinstitutionalisation between the two areas.

Colonies focused on re-training, employment and social care, in particular training colonists for a life of agricultural labour in the countryside.[8] They were founded in part to mitigate the effect of people with epilepsy falling through the gaps between services (the Poor Law, hospitals, asylums and charities) and to provide residential education for children under the age of sixteen.[9] In addition to providing accommodation and training, the colonies were sites of extensive research into epilepsy, and the ability to control environmental factors which were thought to influence severity or frequency of seizures (including medicine, diet, routine and social relationships). Young people's experience within the colonies illustrates a change in scientific understanding of epilepsy, including those related to personality, trauma, stigma and a broad conception of 'stress'. Part of this experience, it will be argued, was an understanding of how the process of enforced transition—the experience of moving between services with nowhere else to go—could have a severe influence on the 'healthy' minds of colony residents.

Social Stigma and Stress in the Colonies

The language used to describe the 'epileptic personality' was similar to that used to describe maladjusted children and was rooted in Freudian psychoanalytic theory. Freud's influence on epilepsy had up to the mid-1930s been on the interpretation of seizures as a form of hysteria. Hysteria and neurasthenia were different from epilepsy in that the seizures presented as something that the patient could control, where the patient did not bite their tongue or fall completely unconscious.[10] Even in the early twentieth century, cases were still being presented in Maida Vale Hospital for Neurology and Neurosurgery which were diagnosed as being hysterical in nature, due in part to the psychological or emotional root of the first seizure.[11] The belief in 'fright' as a cause of seizures altered the perception of people with epilepsy as being born with a disposition that was connected directly to their epilepsy. It suggested that even without direct hereditary factors, people could develop epilepsy following an emotional or psychological shock. Consequently, epilepsy fell between neurology, psychiatry and, later, psychology, in its diagnosis and treatment.

Following the First World War, many neurologists who had been key figures in the treatment of shell shock also developed an interest in epilepsy, such as William Aldren Turner. The psychological and neurological knowledge which resulted in the study of shell shock influenced the medical directors of the colonies. In 1920, Tylor Fox wrote:

> There are a large number of people who are declared epileptics, suffering from fits; and a number more who are potential epileptics, ready to develop fits if they are exposed to severe mental or physical strain. Thus many potential epileptics became actual epileptics under the strain of active service in the European War.[12]

In addition to severe mental and physical strain in later life, epilepsy could be worsened by childhood experiences. Epileptic colonies intended to provide a therapy based on overall well-being. As the first annual report for the Chalfont Colony, run by the National Society for the Employment of Epileptics, noted:

> It is, in the view of the Committee, a matter of primary importance that everyone received at the Colony should be happy and contented, and, as the welfare of the Colony will always depend very largely upon the effects of the Colonists themselves, it is earnestly hoped that all Colonists will endeavour by industry, good temper, cheerfulness, and mutual kindness and forbearance to promote the happiness and well-being of the whole community.[13]

The focus on community living was part of the colony's purpose. This was steeped in a wider context of modernity and anti-modernity, with a strong emphasis on colonists returning to the countryside. In this way, colonists were more closely aligned to open air schools, or collective living, than asylums. Walls were permeable, admission voluntary, and treatment was designed to improve the whole self, rather than merely reduce the rate of seizures. In doing so, the colonies aimed to prevent long-term residency and to support people with epilepsy to find employment outside the colony.

The focus on unemployment stemmed from the colonies' foundation as a means to alleviate urban poverty, in particular casual or precarious labour. Due to the highly variable nature of seizures, and the stigma and danger faced by many people with epilepsy in the industrial workplace, the colonies were initially designed as a means to provide stable, stigma-free employment.[14] Unlike other services, such as work colonies, specialist epileptic colonies explicitly tied the provision of stable work with a reduction in anxiety. An article in *The Lancet* noted:

> The problem of unemployment was widespread and less easy to deal with. The whole question could be regarded as one of mental ill health. Continued unemployment, resentment and anxiety increased the fits, and increase of fits caused further mental deterioration. A vicious circle was set up with the destruction of personality as the end.[15]

This drew a further explicit link between the experience of epilepsy and the experience of stigma, and its consequent effect on mental health, or self-image (described above as 'the destruction of personality'). For children and young people, this was especially pertinent. Tylor Fox wrote extensively from the Lingfield Colony of the difficulties faced by people, especially children, surviving outside the colony:

> From the time of onset of the fits the epileptic member of the household is regarded as someone abnormal, and if, as so often happens, he shows mental peculiarities in addition to the fits, this impression of abnormality is strengthened [...] An epileptic child is not wanted at Church, Chapel or Sunday School, at picture shows or other entertainments. The parents, bothered by having him repeatedly brought home after fits in the street, or naturally anxious about his safety from accident, tend to keep the child more and more within doors, with disastrous results to his health.[16]

Unlike the stigma faced outside the colony, the colonies aimed to provide a safe and secure environment for its residents. In effect, the colonists' entire world within the colony walls was subject to scrutiny and prescription. For some, this had good results, with a doctor in Pennsylvania noting that 'all patients now at the colony are distinctly improved in physical and mental health, and in a large majority there is a marked reduction in the number and severity of attacks'.[17] This was echoed in the 1895 Annual Report for the National Society for the Employment of Epileptics, the governing body of the Chalfont Colony in Buckinghamshire, that stated, 'The improvement in the general well-being of the Colonists has been most encouraging, and it is far greater than can be measured by the mere diminution in the frequency and severity of fits'.[18]

Unlike other colonies, the David Lewis Centre in Manchester stated in its first Annual Report that the aim was not to reduce seizures, but to improve the overall well-being of its inhabitants—regardless of whether they had more or fewer seizures.[19] According to the 1912 Report of the Chief Medical Officer of the Board of Education, most children with epilepsy attended regular mainstream school. In cases where they did not, attendance at a special residential school was due to a number of factors, not all relating to the frequency or severity of seizures. In some cases, the child had been excluded from school following a seizure, or following a period of inattentiveness, hyperactivity or poor attendance.[20] Quoting the neurologist David Ferrier, the Report noted that this was due to 'the occurrence of fits in a school causes all kinds of nervous disturbances on the part of other children, and the terror sometimes caused by epilepsy might induce it in others who had a predisposition…the whole school may be upset in consequence'.[21] Yet, Ferrier argued epilepsy itself was not a reason for children not to attend school. He wrote:

> I do not see apart from [the fear of other children] why epileptics should not be educated with other children, so far as their mental condition is concerned. Some are very clever. Many persons occupying responsible positions in society are suffering from epilepsy and are doing excellent work.[22]

The primary concern of the authorities was that children's epilepsy was a source of fear for other people—necessitating exclusion of these children from wider society. This was argued by Ferrier to benefit the child, also, whose confidence and ability were said to improve once he or she was in a situation which allowed 'lively intercourse with other children' rather than exclusion.[23] As a result, the Defective and Epileptic Children Act put measures into place which provided a requirement for residential schools to be set up, linked with epileptic colonies.[24] The Board of Education noted that:

> A young epileptic child stands a better chance of arrest if taken in hand as soon as the fits declare themselves. It is detrimental to the young epileptic to keep it at home, where it becomes spoiled, remains uneducated, and where the chance of arrest from fits is deterred through petting and inadequate medical and open-air training.[25]

Even those who were against institutionalisation of children believed that the case of children with epilepsy was different. When in a community where seizures were the norm, children with epilepsy were enabled to reach their full potential, without fear of social isolation or exclusion. The irony of this was the same as other residential care schemes—in order for the children not to experience social isolation, the children were required to be cut off from mainstream society. M. K. Inglis argued in the *Fortnightly Review* in 1908 that removing children from the homes of poor families was detrimental to the long-term development of children as they lacked the stability and love that their family should be able to provide. Inglis wrote that 'no institution system, however perfect nor "Home", however few the number of inmates it contains, can make up for the loss of the rough-and-tumble of family life, and for father and mother and sister and brother love'.[26] Inglis noted, however, the special social status of the child with epilepsy:

> There are, however, certain classes of children who *must* be taken from their homes and kept under special conditions if the best is to be made of their own lives, and if a healthy life is to be made possible for the other members of the family; such are most cases of epileptic and mentally defective children. For them the danger of the streets is manifold, and they require very special training and protection long after they cease to be children.[27]

Fifty years later, in 1962, de Haas reiterated that children with epilepsy faced social stigma. The stigma originated from teachers who lacked knowledge of seizures and lived in fear of a child experiencing a seizure in front of their classmates. Often, the fear other children experienced, in addition to the isolation felt by the child, was the main barrier for attending mainstream school.[28] As with other aspects of life, only if the child was able to 'mask' their epilepsy would they be accepted socially. This in itself was thought to have a profound impact on the emotional state of the child—increasing their fear of seizures and impacting on their mental health.

Epilepsy and the Family Home

In 1906, William Gowers argued that epilepsy was often prevalent in families with a history of insanity or alcoholism. In addition to viewing these as inherited illnesses, Fox identified the impact that this environment may have on a child with epilepsy. He noted in 1920 that 'the parents themselves so often show evidences of mental instability[...] evidences of minor mental derangement, whether they come under the heading of hysteria, neurasthenia, violent tempers or addiction to drugs are likely to be prevalent also'.[29] He gave the example of a case where a girl aged twelve years old experienced violence at the hands of her parents, involving violent tempers 'which sometimes result[ed] in crockery flying about'.[30] Although Fox attributed some hereditary factors to the family's history of mental illness, Fox noted 'it is difficult to think of an atmosphere in which [seizures] are less likely to be controlled'.[31]

Ralph Crowley's work on 'the social care of the epileptic' examined the rates of 'broken homes' among children with epilepsy, noting that in two cases out of sixty the child's epilepsy was thought to be the cause of the separation.[32] Reiterating Fox's findings, Crowley noted that in many of the cases, the prevalence of 'homes in which a parent was psychoneurotic had some form of mental illness was particularly high'.[33] Therefore, it was not only the influence of wider society on the child's psychological experience, but the experience in this home. The psychological impact of this was believed to have an effect on the number and frequency of seizures, and highlighted a growing discourse not only of the impact of stigma on mental health, but the impact of poor mental health on seizure frequency.

The social stigma experienced by children with epilepsy was not confined exclusively to their experience of seizures, but also to their experience of being 'an epileptic' and the impact this had on a chaotic family life. Part of this was the construction of the 'epileptic personality', where a set of negative personality traits or behaviours were attributed to children who had seizures. An unknown author in *The Lancet* noted:

> There is general agreement that epileptics, as a class, are more egocentric and more sensitive than the rest of the community-that they are poor in ideas and unstable in their emotions. Thus they are said to possess the epileptic personality.[34]

This 'epileptic personality' was seen as the lesser form of the criminal epileptic. The epileptic personality suggested the potential for violence or uncontrollability and became further associated with poverty and delinquency. The family, and the child's place within the family, became synonymous with the child's place within society. The case of Robert, a patient in Craig Colony, NY, demonstrates the connectivity between chaotic lives, urban poverty, and an 'epileptic temperament'. Robert's case notes reported that he was raised by his mother (an alcoholic of 'loose morals'), an uncle who taught him to steal, and his father who could not afford to care for him. After being abandoned by his mother, Robert was transferred into foster care in Long Island, yet gained a juvenile record and was transferred to Randall's Island, an institution for feeble-minded children in New York at the age of twelve. Robert's personality was recorded in detail during the mental examination:

> As a personality, he already displays the epileptic make-up. He has a poverty of interests other than those directly related to himself, he is egotistic, refuses to play basketball with team work and is expelled. Unemotional, set forth by the teachers has no ideas of the rights of others. In addition to his personality of epileptic traits he presents as a psychopathic type of delinquent.[35]

By the 1960s, the influence of the Child Guidance movement and attachment theory was added to Freudian ideas of parental influence. Central to this was the parent–child relationship, and the role that the child's epilepsy played in the development or stunting of that relationship. Inter-family relationships were complex, and the position of epilepsy within these relationships was seen to be no different from any other personality trait or attribute. In this way, the child's epilepsy could either be part of the parent–child conflict or else the basis for a parent's reaction to the child. This in itself served as a reason for removing children from the home, noting that when removed from these parental conflicts, a child could thrive. As Lorentz de Haas, from the Meer en Bosch Epilepsy Centre in the Netherlands, wrote in 1962:

> There are conditions under which the epileptic seizure becomes a weapon for the child in a difficult family situation, in which the seizure is integrated in a neuropathic defence system, or in which, in reverse, the child's epilepsy becomes a psychological necessity to the family, as a result of which a cure is unconsciously sabotaged. [...] in 17 children with petit mal epilepsy found an impaired parent-child relationship as a cause. In every instance there was a conscious parental rejection with attending overt hostility or unconscious parental rejection with attending compensatory overprotection and thinly veiled hostility.[36]

The colony institution aimed to re-create the family atmosphere, but away from the chaotic or detrimental aspects of domestic conflict. In addition to removing the child from an environment of stigma or isolation, the colony could provide stability, which would prevent maladjustment:

> Although during his stay in the institution, the child is somewhat more remote from normal society, we believe that personality development during a given period in relative peace can sometimes better prepare this

> personality for meeting the exigencies of later life in society. Because epileptic children rather often come from disturbed homes, it must also be remarked that they can lead "a sensible and stable life" in the epilepsy centres and colonies, away from their homes.[37]

Stress, childhood trauma and poor home life were often referred to as the cause of seizures, and the daily life at the colony was aimed to mitigate other triggers, such as heat. Residential schools offered medical superintendents the opportunity to draw links between seizure frequency among the children in schools and environmental surroundings. The logbook for the Soss Moss School (run by the Manchester Education Authority) frequently reported the weather as a cause of an unusual increase in the frequency of seizures in the classroom. In June 1903, the head–teacher noted, 'The weather has been hot and thundery during the week and it seems to have had considerable effect on the health of the children, they seem to be more liable to fits'.[38] Two weeks later, it was again noted, 'the hot weather however appears to affect some of the children so as to make them restless and to make them more liable to fits'.[39] This understanding of the physical environment's impact on the mental health of the children further demonstrates how the twentieth century saw a diversification in the understanding of the experience and causes of epilepsy. Clearly removing children from their family home was just the first step in removing these children from the stresses of daily life and inculcating a philosophy of healthy minds.

Colonies and After-Care

The Education (Defective and Epileptic Children) Act, 1899 ensured that local authorities provided residential care and education for children with epilepsy. The Act stipulated that children would be under the remit of the Act until they were sixteen years old. This was above the leaving age of mainstream education, yet significantly below the average age of adult entries to the colonies. Colony schools were set up with the aim of either educating children for mainstream capital-labour markets, or else preparing them for colony life, significant amount of emphasis was placed on the outcomes of children upon leaving the colonies. This differed in the UK and the United States. In the UK, the emphasis was placed on the employment prospects of post-colony life. Advocates like Tylor Fox extensively studied this vulnerable period, campaigning for more social care for young people with epilepsy.[40] This may, in fact, be one of the central reasons why Lingfield's legacy lay in the creation of a charity specifically aimed at the rights and abilities of young people with epilepsy.[41] In the UK, the design of the colonies meant that young people were expected to stay for significantly longer. Yet, many people left, due either to parents removing them (in the case of voluntary patients) or else being removed after parents obtained a court order.[42]

Epileptic colonies shared similar characteristics to post-war therapeutic communities, in particular their belief that treatment should be holistic, with the focus on the self.[43] In the UK, the colonies were a short-term solution. The colony provided education, training and medical care so that colonists would leave and becoming sufficient. For this to be successful, the colony needed to integrate itself with community medical settings so that work began at the colony would continue. In 1920, Hume Griffiths, medical director of the Lingfield Colony, noted:

> [The children leaving colony schools] have been carefully looked after for years, even had their games organised, only be to pitch-forked into the outside world, to sink or swim […] when the age of sixteen is reached, [any] responsibility ceases and, unless he or she can be transferred to a Board of Guardians, the child is withdrawn, lives in unsuitable surroundings, the treatment is stopped, often suddenly.[44]

Griffiths highlighted that this enforced transition between the colony and the outside world, or between the colony and other services, had a profound impact on the mental health of young people with epilepsy. In 1921, Tylor Fox made several references to the link between stress, anxiety and seizures. While the routine of the colony served to reduce this stress by providing education, a stable home and employment, there were some instances where the colony itself often produced anxiety in its inhabitants. He noted:

> In my experience one of the most potent factors in producing fits in one liable to them is continual worry or apprehension. When an epileptic child has some fear or anxiety on his mind, it seems almost useless to expect any improvement until that anxiety is removed. We have often noticed at Lingfield that as a child approaches his sixteenth birthday, and realises that we are deciding whether he must stay on the colony or be allowed to return home, his fits increase in number.[45]

Through their analysis of enforced transitions, Fox and Hume Griffiths drew a direct link not only between transition and poor mental health, but between poor mental health and an increase in seizures. This, in turn, reflected a growing understanding that epilepsy was not only in the remit of neurologists, but required a more comprehensive and holistic approach to treatment.

Colony after-care therefore became a key area of discussion among those working in epilepsy medical and social research. The lack of information on the outcomes of children leaving residential care was due in part to the difficulty in following-up cases. As the Chief Medical Officer of the Board of Education noted in 1912, this could be improved by 'a closer association between the authorities of the residential institutions and the school medical officers and any after-care committee from whom the children are received'.[46] Individual colony schools made some attempt to trace its alumni. In 1907, Soss Moss School, run by the Manchester Education Authority, yet tied to the David Lewis Colony, reported the end of the school career for children in the following two entries:

> [One boy] who was admitted on Dec 13th last left the school on Saturday as he was sixteen years of age. He will remain in the adult part of the colony. [one girl] who has been here for over two years left today. She has not had any 'attack' since she came. She is intelligent but inclines to be careless about the way she does things.[47]

In November of the same year, the logbook reported another two cases:

> One boy [...] left on Monday last, 28th inst. He was over 16 years of age; he has gone to the adult part of the Colony. He has been here nearly a year and a half. He had made good progress in reading, but he was very babyish in many respects and very weak minded.[48]
>
> [...] leaves tomorrow to go to the adult part of the Colony. For many months he got no benefit from being in school. Most of the time he sat in his desk without giving the last attention to what was going on with the class. Occasionally he had brief interest, when he was eager to take part in the class work, but as a rule he had to be left to do nothing.[49]

Many reports were given of young people aged sixteen who were seen as not progressing in the colony schools. The head–teacher (author of the report) noted frequently that many of the pupils in the colony school were mentally not capable of benefiting from the colony education. For many of them, this meant being transferred to the adult section of the [David Lewis] colony in order to remain for a longer period of time. These young people were in a manner of speaking the 'failure' of the colony; although admitted, presumably, as sane or mentally developed, many of the young people presented symptoms of advanced deterioration.

In 1916, Hume Griffith attempted to trace school leavers from Lingfield. He contacted local authorities and received information on 80 ex-colony residents in order to produce an after-care report, the majority of whom had left the colony within four years. Out of these, 22% were 'wholly or partially self-sufficient'. Griffiths noted that for this section, many had been removed from the colony against medical advice, as 'parents insist on parental rights'. The 'sufficiency' of those in this section was due to the cessation of seizures, which, Griffiths noted, was likely to be temporary. Those 'partially self-sufficient' were unlikely to be in work, due to 'fear of the Workman's Compensation Act'.[50] Of those that were employed, one was employed in a shop, six in the army, eleven not mentioned, one handyman and one in the chemical works. Griffiths noted that 'at present they take any job that offers, and go from one situation to another'.[51] This pattern was also seen at Starnthwaite, Lingfield's sister colony, where the vast majority of leavers from 1905 to 1913 (ranging in ages from 14 to 24) were transferred to the adult part of the colony and employed as farm labourers. For those transferred to the adult colony, 'mental weakness' often led to subsequent transfers to workhouse or infirmaries. In a few cases, employment was gained outside an institutional setting. In one case, the person was 'in partnership with a brother as a decorator and signwriter'. In another case, a person was described as, 'able to assist a little in the printing office' despite still having seizures, yet another was 'taken home by parents on reaching age limit, working at a market gardener's earning 10s a week'.[52] This data was perhaps influenced by gender, with the population of Starnthwaite's school leavers being boys. Records for both Maghull Colony and school leavers in the Leicester district demonstrate that a higher number of girls remained at home in the care of parents, with boys being more likely to be maintained in an adult colony or under the care of the Board of Guardians.[53] This was due to economic patterns, as male leavers were able to gain precarious employment as labourers and were more likely (on a whole population level) to have higher earning power. The colony, therefore, merely offered temporary respite from the precarious labour market and stigma faced outside the institution's walls. The enforced transition for those school leavers was a stark cliff-edge between security inside the colony and precarity and stigma outside it.

For the most part, those transferred to the adult colony were transferred not on the basis of their mental capacity (though, these cases are from before the regular usage of intelligence testing). For many, it was the absence of self-sufficiency being demonstrated, either in their ability to perform tasks or in their communication or response to social cues. In the above cases, limited concentration or engagement with the colony school curriculum was enough to demonstrate to the school authorities that any young person was not only unfit for school life, but for life in the 'outside world'. For their post-colony life to be successful, young people needed not only to demonstrate a life free from seizures, but to demonstrate a certain attitude, personality and work ethic. The young people resident in Soss Moss School followed the same pattern as those in Lingfield:

> Lizzie M(-) who was sixteen years of age on the 17th inst left school yesterday. She is not free from occasional epileptic fits but she is otherwise strong and healthy, fairly intelligent and under suitable supervision would be very useful in domestic work. She is good at needlework.[54]

For many young people, success outside the colony depended on a combination of personality, health and available support. In effect, young people as with the cases above had to demonstrate that they were 'useful'. In the same vein, colony proponents, educators and medical officers also had to demonstrate that the colony system could produce 'useful' people. For those that had little chance, the adult colonies were a final reserve. If unable to work, or to be self-sufficient, and (for many) in the absence of friends and relatives, transfer to the adult colony meant an escape albeit temporarily from the workhouse and asylum or homelessness. The familiarity of the colonies often meant that those transferred to the adult colonies would often from the age of sixteen have worked and lived with their future home-mates, creating minimal upheaval in the transition from school to adult life.

The nature of the epileptic colonies was that adults who were admitted were there for a long duration. Young people, however, were there to attend school, after which they were expected to find employment. Fox's extensive efforts to maintain a link between the children's and the adults' sections of the colonies led to further research into the transition between services, both between the colony and the community and between hospital departments and other services outside the colony. As Ralph Crowley, former senior medical officer to the Board of Education wrote in the Lancet in 1938:

> The hospital doctor, the private practitioner, the mental welfare worker, and the aftercare visitor acting as a team and backed by the community could bring untold relief to the daily lot of the epileptic. Such a welfare organization must operate early if it is to prevent the maladjustments of adult epileptics.[55]

In 1948, the National Committee for Mental Health had a dedicated Committee for Epileptics, which was tasked with implementing measures to improve the lives of people with epilepsy. As reported in *Epilepsia*, one of these measures was the introduction of hostels, or halfway stations, between the hospital and the community. These hostels aimed to provide the kind of employment provided in the epileptic colonies, but maintain a close relationship with outpatient departments and mainstream services. In addition, the Committee made reports to the Under Secretary of Labour that special clinics be set up for people with epilepsy 'with an emphasis on social and vocational aspects'.[56] By the mid-twentieth century, then, services for people with epilepsy recognised not only the strong psychological component of seizures, but the impact of enforced transitions between services.

Conclusions

For children who were considered to have an 'epileptic personality', the colonies were a respite from chaotic homes and social stigma. Robert, a resident at the Craig Colony, was moved frequently from house to locked ward to house, both gaining and losing responsibility dependent on behaviour. Throughout this time, the boy's reports were largely positive, with staff at the colony noting that he was charismatic, intelligent and got on well with many attendants. Some years after absconding from the colony, he wrote to the superintendent:

> I ran away from Sonyea because I could only see my father once a year and it would cost him a whole lot to go from NYC to Sonyea […] I am in one of the biggest hospitals of N.Y and it is a lunatic asylum. That is the

> nearest an epileptic can get to his locality hear [sic] in NYC [...] two years ago my father passed off. I am now 30 sitting among full lunatics watching walls, with no freedom we had on Sonyea.[57]

Up to 1965, a growing body of research examined the ways in which the experience of social stigma and family conflicts could have an effect on seizures, largely by creating an environment of stress and insecurity for young people. The colonies were seen as places of stability, where young people were able to feel at home and where they were protected from the conflicts of the family. Yet, at age sixteen, many young people were no longer offered accommodation or support, and the enforced transition between the colony and the outside world often caused poor mental health and an increase in seizures. This led to a move towards greater integration of services, with an emphasis on social care as well as medical care. This association between stress and seizures was not necessarily new, but it did demonstrate that the treatment in the colonies had moved away from a general belief in the benefits of fresh air, exercise and diet (that which categories most asylum regimes at the time) and instead created a direct and causal link between anxiety and seizures.

The psychosocial experience of epilepsy enabled the history of epilepsy to be viewed within a wider history of mental health. This has a particular significance for the political position of epilepsy within the disability studies movement. As is the case with epilepsy services, the study of epilepsy also necessarily has to cross the bridge between neurology and psychiatry. People with epilepsy often categorise their psychosocial experience as one of fear: both the fear of seizures and the fear of being 'found out' or unmasked. For a large part of the twentieth century, this fear was based on the social reality of isolation, of 'being epileptic' and the necessity of creating a whole new social enclave in which children were able to thrive. The International League Against Epilepsy's emphasis on childhood experiences and stigma drew the discussion of epilepsy away from a medical model and towards a psychosocial model of seizures. As Rhodes et al. noted, this in itself highlights the importance of the social model of disability and the history of social oppression experienced by people with epilepsy. Yet, the historical need to protect mental health through a process of masking often led to an unwillingness to self-identify as disabled.

Notes

1. Owsei Temkin, *The Falling Sickness: A History of Epilepsy from the Greeks to the Beginnings of Modern Neurology* (Baltimore: John Hopkins University Press, 1994).
2. Penny Rhodes, Andrew Nocon, Neil Small, and John Wright, "Disability and Identity: The Challenge of Epilepsy." *Disability & Society* 23, no. 4 (June 2008): 385–395.
3. Erving Goffman, *Stigma: Notes on the Management of Spoiled Identity* (Harmondsworth: Penguin Books, 1968).
4. G. E. Berrios, *Insanity and Epilepsy in the Nineteenth Century* (London: Gaskell Press, 1979).
5. Hedi Rimke and Alan Hunt, "From Sinners to Degenerates: The Medicalization of Morality in the Late Nineteenth Century." *History of the Human Sciences* 15, no. 1 (2002): 59–89, 71; Anita Rogan, *Perceptions of Epilepsy in the Second Half of the Nineteenth Century* (MSc Thesis, Wellcome Library, 1993).
6. Mervyn J. Eadie, *A Disease Once Sacred: A History of the Medical Understanding of Epilepsy*, ed. Peter F. Bladin (Eastleigh: John Libbey, 2001); Diana P. Faber, "Jean-Martin Charcot and the Epilepsy/Hysteria Relationship." *Journal of the History of the Neurosciences* 6, no. 3 (December 1997): 275–290.
7. E. Thornton, *Hypnotism, Hysteria and Epilepsy: An Historical Synthesis* (London: Heinemann Medical, 1976).
8. Jean Barclay, *The First Epileptic Home in England: A Centenary History of the Maghull Homes 1888–1988* (Glasgow: Heatherbank Press, 1990); Jean Barclay, *Langho Colony, Langho Centre, 1906–1984: A Contextual Study of Manchester's Public Institution for People with Epilepsy* (Manchester: Manchester Social Services, 1989).
9. Rachel Hewitt, "Lingfield Training Centre, Work Colonies and the Development of Specialist Care for People with Epilepsy 1890–1902." *Postgraduate Journal of Medical Humanities* 3 (2016): 2–23.
10. Peter F. Bladin, "Historical Note: 'The Epileptic Constitution': The Psychoanalytic Concept of Epilepsy." *Journal of the History of Neurosciences* 9, no. 1 (August 2000): 94.
11. Queen Square Library, NHNN/CN/2/3 Jackson and Gowers Case Book (1879), 21. Also reported by William Gowers, a case where a young boy was frightened in violent robbery, who reported seeing the flash of a knife before his seizures.
12. Joseph Tylor Fox, *The Care of Sane Epileptic Children* (London: J. Bale, 1920).

13. London Metropolitan Archives [Hereafter LMA] A/FWA/D/D128/1 "Life at the Colony" pamphlet, Charity Organisation Society Correspondence (c. 1900).
14. Hewitt, "Lingfield Training Centre," 2–23.
15. New York State Archives [Hereafter NYSA] B1901 Superintendent's memoranda c. 1901–1935, cutting from Unknown Author, "The Place of Epileptics in the Community." *The Lancet* (28 November 1936): 1291.
16. Fox, *The Care of Sane Epileptic Children*, 21.
17. NYSA, B1901 Superintendent's memoranda c. 1901–1935, cutting from Charles Letchworth c. 1930.
18. LMA, A/FWA/D/D128/1 "Report of the Honourable Medical Secretary to the Chalfont Colony," Chalfont Colony Annual Report (1895).
19. University of Manchester Library GB 133 MMC/9/42 David Lewis Epileptic Colony, Annual Report (1905) Aims and Objectives.
20. Board of Education, *Annual Report for 1912 of the Chief Medical Officer of the Board of Education* (London: Wyman and Sons, 1913), 108.
21. Ibid., 47.
22. Ibid., 27–28.
23. Ibid., 29.
24. The National Archives [Hereafter TNA], ED 50/271 Board of Education Minute Paper, Dr. Eichholtz and Dr. Crowley Revision of Articles 22 and 23 of the Special Schools Regulation (1914).
25. TNA, ED 50/271 Discussion of the Minute of the Board of Education dated 15th February 1918 modifying the regulations for Special Schools (i.e. schools for Blind, Deaf, Defective and Epileptic children).
26. M. K. Inglis, "The State Versus the Home." *Fortnightly Review* 84, no. 502 (1908): 643–659, 647.
27. Ibid.
28. A. M. Lorentz de Haas, "Social Aspects of Epilepsy in Childhood." *Epilepsia* 3, no. 1 (March 1962): 44–55, 47.
29. Fox, *The Care of Sane Epileptic Children*, 21.
30. Ibid.
31. Ibid.
32. Ralph H. Crowley, "The Social Care of the Epileptic." *The Lancet* (1936): 61–64.
33. Ibid., 62.
34. Unknown Author, "The Epileptic Personality." *The Lancet* (1934): 1400.
35. NYSA, Albany, NY, B2749-13 Craig Colony Case Books, Box 12 Case 4912 c. 1918.
36. Lorentz de Haas, "Social Aspects of Epilepsy," 46.
37. Crowley, "The Social Care of the Epileptic," 61–64.
38. Soss Moss Log Book, 3rd June 1903, Records of the Soss Moss School, Manchester Education Authority, Manchester Record Office.

39. Ibid., 24 June.
40. A. Hume Griffith and G. Savage, "After-Care Report of Epileptics following Colony Treatment." *British Journal of Psychiatry* (1916): 151–167.
41. "Celebrating 118 Years at Young Epilepsy," [online] Young Epilepsy. Accessed 18 December 2019. http://www.youngepilepsy.org.uk/news-and-events/news/celebrating-118-years-at-young-epilepsy.html.
42. See NYSA, Craig Colony Clinical Records.
43. Frederick B. Glaser, "Some Historical Aspects of the Drug-Free Therapeutic Community." *The American Journal of Drug and Alcohol Abuse* 1, no. 1 (1974): 37–52; Nick Crossley, "Working Utopias and Social Movements: An Investigation Using Case Study Materials from Radical Mental Health Movements in Britain." *Sociology* 33, no. 4 (1999): 809–830.
44. Ibid., 155.
45. Fox, *The Care of Sane Epileptic Children*, 130.
46. Report of the Medical Officer of the Board of Education, 1912, 108.
47. Manchester Record Office M66/40/1/1/1/ David Lewis Colony School (Soss Moss School) log book, 31.
48. Ibid., 38.
49. Ibid., 39.
50. Griffith and Savage, 'After-Care Report," 151–167.
51. Ibid., 152.
52. Report of the Medical Officer of the Board of Education (1912), 126–127.
53. Ibid., 125.
54. Soss Moss Log Book, 51.
55. Crowley, "The Social Care of the Epileptic."
56. Dennis Williams, "The British League Against Epilepsy." *Epilepsia* 3, no. 4 (December 1948): 272–274, 272.
57. NYSA, Albany, NY, B2749-13 Craig Colony Case Books, Box 12 Case 4912 c. 1918.

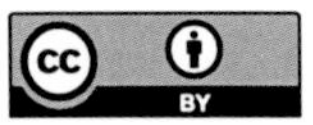
BY

CHAPTER 4

Planning for the Future: Special Education and the Creation of 'Healthy Minds'

Steven J. Taylor

Introduction

This chapter turns to explore how special education developed in England to manage a population of children living with mental impairment. Focusing primarily on the years following the introduction of the Education Act (Epileptic and Defective Children), 1899, it explores the identification, observation, certification and methods of 'managing' those deemed to not be mentally healthy enough to attend mainstream or, as they were referred to historically, 'ordinary' schools. The influence of government legislation and regulatory bodies alongside the local experience of special education at the Sandwell Hall School for Mentally Defective Children, near Birmingham, is to be considered. Furthermore, it will examine the level of professionalisation and expertise that emerged among those managing the school. The chapter thus seeks to deal with abstract conceptualisations of 'healthy' minds, as well as more tangible lived experiences.

S. J. Taylor (✉)
School of History, University of Leicester, Leicester, UK
e-mail: sjt48@leicester.ac.uk

S. J. Taylor and A. Brumby (eds.), *Healthy Minds in the Twentieth Century*, Mental Health in Historical Perspective,
https://doi.org/10.1007/978-3-030-27275-3_4

Special education at this time was embedded in legislative policy and a broader socio-medical discourse. Mathew Thomson has argued that the beginning of the twentieth century was a turning point when society came to see itself through a 'psychological' prism. Such a transformation had particular implications for children as they passed through the mainstream elementary education system and its psychology influenced pedagogy.[1] Ordinary schools began to offer a more child-centred approach to the curriculum at this time, which may have been more frustrating and less accessible for children with learning difficulties than the learning by memory and discipline of the nineteenth-century schoolroom. The special school thus was markedly different from the ordinary school.

Mark Jackson has conducted an in-depth study of Mary Dendy and the Sandlebridge School that she founded in Cheshire for mentally defective children.[2] In his work, Jackson uses this school as a prism to gain a more thorough insight into ideas about 'feeble-mindedness' at the end of the nineteenth century. Dendy believed that mental deficiency lay at the root of social problems and subsequently she promoted the permanent segregation of the mentally deficient individual for their own good and that of society.[3] Like Jackson's work, this chapter uses a special school as a lens for its analysis but in a very different way. Here we delve more into the mechanics of special education through the experience of the Sandwell School for Mentally Defective Children, to examine issues of education, charity, policy and, to a degree, lived experience, whereas Jackson considered ideas about the nature of feeble-mindedness and how they were shaped by institutional experience.

As we find elsewhere in this volume, particularly the contributions from Jan Walmsley and Michelle O'Reilly et al., defining and classifying mental illness and disability have been important areas of discussion. In this chapter, classification is a particularly fluid issue as the Education Act (Epileptic and Mentally Defective Children), 1899, did not define the criteria for determining 'defectiveness' and the later Mental Deficiency Act, 1913, served as social rather than educational legislation.[4] The measure applied in practice was the ability to benefit from education, but not being mentally disabled or 'merely dull or backward'.[5] Subsequently, there was a degree of subjectivity related to the type of children that were admitted to special schools, and Pamela Dale has observed that 'education was marginalized by other agendas that prioritized long-term care and control'.[6] Subsequently, as we have seen in Rachel Hewitt's chapter dealing with the work of epileptic colonies, this was a contested area that focused on developing mentally defective children for independent adult lives but also, if necessary, preparing them for a lifetime of care and control in specialised institutions.

These spaces of care were almost as ill-defined as the types of individuals they were built to accommodate. Looking at the Birmingham area more specifically, Rebecca Wynter, using the Monyhull Epileptic Colony as a lens, emphasises the importance of local lay individuals such as Ellen Pinsent, who features in more depth later in this chapter, in the process of identifying and separating 'unhealthy' minds from the healthy.[7] Wynter concludes that definitions of mental defectiveness operated at local levels despite often being enshrined in national legislation. Therefore, when assessing the experience of the Sandwell Hall School in this chapter, both local and national definitions of healthy minds will be presented.

Legislating for Healthy Minds

Twentieth-century concerns about the intellectual abilities of children have their roots in the second half of the previous century. The Lunacy Acts of 1845 legislated on a mass-scale for the compulsory confinement and treatment of England's insane population in publicly funded lunatic asylums. Yet, while there have been numerous scholarly studies that have explored the nature of institutional confinement for the insane,[8] children have received less attention.[9] In the fifty years following the Lunacy Acts the number of people, children included, in Britain certified as a 'lunatic', 'imbecile' or 'idiot' exploded. It was estimated that by 1909 there were 271,000 certified lunatics and mentally defectives in England and Wales, 'or very nearly one in every 100 of the population'.[10] Despite the mass building of asylums and workhouse lunacy wards, authorities and doctors were ill-equipped to offer effective treatment to such large numbers.[11] Subsequently, mental illness and disability became increasingly important issues at a national level.

Coinciding with changing attitudes towards mental health, children, as a distinct population, also emerged as a specific concern of policymakers, reformers and philanthropists in the second half of the nineteenth century.[12] Ideas of national efficiency and potential imperial decline were the driving force behind these changes. The young, and particularly the offspring of the urban working poor, were increasingly depicted as the future of both nation and empire within these discourses.

As the first Chief Medical Officer at the Board of Education, George Newman, observed 'children determine the destinies of all civilisations, that the race or society which succeeds with its mammoth ships and its manufactures but fails to produce men and women, is on the brink of irretrievable doom'.[13] At a national level, there was an increased focus on children, placing value on their education and the removal of factors detrimental to their development. Importantly, for the themes of this volume, there was a belief in the contaminating influence of unhealthy minds, which led to the segregation of those with learning disabilities from the mainstream school population. The academic capabilities of 'deficient' and 'defective' children thus were linked directly to the social and economic potential of the nation.

These concerns led to a sustained medical interest in the training and management of children with supposedly unhealthy minds. Perhaps the most influential voice in this area was Dr. George E. Shuttleworth who worked as Assistant Medical Officer at the Earlswood Idiot Asylum and Medical Superintendent at the Royal Albert Asylum. In 1895, Shuttleworth published, what he described as, a 'little Manual to the Medical Profession, and to the increasing number of the Public who take an interest in the special education of mentally deficient children'.[14] Aware of his professional and lay audience the 'manual' spanned an array of issues including social context, medical classification, aetiology, treatment and education, while attempting to discuss gradations of impairment from the 'dull' to 'idiots', who were considered to be the most severe of cases.[15] The section on education is most relevant to this chapter and volume. Shuttleworth subdivided this into three sections: 'educational', 'industrial' and 'moral'.[16] Educational training was concerned with the physical and mental development of the child and followed the Froebelian philosophy of learning through doing. There was a focus on 'sensory' training over the 'three R's' that formed the backbone of the mainstream school curriculum. The section on industrial education dealt with activities that could be adopted in special schools that would best prepare children for their adult lives as part of an industrial workforce. Some examples include paper weaving—considered good preparation for the trade of sock darning, and the 'pricker', used for perforated pictures, that was seen as an introduction to cobbling.[17] Of course, many of these activities were gender specific and while boys were guided towards, depending on their ability, carpentry, woodcarving, gardening and farming, girls were 'encouraged to take an interest in domestic matters and to assist in the still-room'.[18] The third strand, moral education, aimed to interweave with the academic and industrial elements of a child's education in order to instil the core pillars of middle-class respectability. There was an underlying belief that the feeble-minded were susceptible to slip into vice and criminality and therefore effective moral education would help to prevent social decline.[19] To reinforce the moral instruction Shuttleworth promoted a system of rewards (such as praise in front of peers and commendation) and punishment (which included corporeal punishment, although the effectiveness was questioned, and withholding favourite foods).[20] Thus, we can see from Shuttleworth's work that shaping young unhealthy minds into future socially efficient and respectable citizens was paramount.

Despite the work and influence of Shuttleworth, debate continued about the nature of mentally deficient children and following the passage of the Mental Deficiency Act in 1913, Alfred Binet and Thomas Simon published their work on intelligence testing in France. Their attention was on children that they defined as 'abnormal' and they explained this classification to mean 'those who are suitable neither for the ordinary school nor the asylum; for the school they are not sufficiently good, for the asylum not sufficiently bad'.[21] It was from this population of supposedly 'abnormal' children that the special schools were populated. Binet and Simon's work was designed to provide an objective and scientific rationale for special education after criticising the subjectivity and 'selfish interests' of philanthropy in establishing the schools.[22] The motives of those managing schools are something that we will turn to later in this chapter. Binet and Simon measured the abilities of an individual to those of a supposedly 'normal' child of the same age and then divided the mental age by the actual age to reveal the intelligence quotient or IQ. According to their formula, children under nine who were two years behind in mental development were 'probably' deficient, and those aged over nine whose development was three years behind were 'definitely' deficient. These tests functioned as a guide to ensure the admission of the correct children to special schools, making sure that those who could progress in an ordinary school, nor those that would not advance in any educational setting did not enter. There was initially a slow take up in England, but the attempt to create an unhealthy mind, as a classification based in science, is an important one.

In Birmingham, the tests were not taken up and the School Board adopted the approach of providing special classes, rather than schools for suitable children. As early as December 1900, all of these had been certified by the Board of Education under the Elementary Education (Defective and Epileptic Children) Act, 1899.[23] To get a sense of demand on these special classes, the School Board of the city, in 1903, commissioned school attendance officers to conduct an analysis of the number of defective children receiving an education. The method of counting was, somewhat, imperfect considering that attendance officers only had contact with children already known to them but the results, in Table 4.1, reveal the range of issues that were dealt with in special classes at the time.[24]

It is immediately evident that children with supposed unhealthy minds numbered fewer than those with physical impairments. However, this was a rudimentary counting exercise that did not take into account the 'invisibility' of mental health issues and the fears that parents might have in disclosing them to authorities, especially if it might bring them closer to requiring medical relief from the much maligned poor law. Furthermore, there is a lack of nuance in the classification system with no insight into how many of those counted as 'weak intellect,

Table 4.1 The prevalence of 'defective' children in Birmingham schools, 1903

	Under 5 years	*5–14 attending school*	*5–14 not attending school*	*Over 14 years*	*Total*
Cripples	24	33	146	0	203
Deaf, deaf and dumb, dumb, or defective speech	3	19	25	2	47
Defective sight	1	4	55	0	60
Epileptics	11	4	39	0	52
St Vitus Dance	0	1	18	0	19
Weak intellect, feeble-minded, imbecile	2	39	61	0	102
Various diseases	0	0	10	0	10
Total	41	98	352	2	493

Source Wolfson Centre for Archival Research, Birmingham Education Committee, Special Schools Committee of the School Board Minutes, 10 February 1898–17 March 1903, SB/B11/1/1/1, p. 214

feeble-minded, and imbecile' would have benefited from education, a key factor in filtering children into the classes. These numbers therefore need to be handled with a healthy degree of cynicism, but are nevertheless useful in providing some context into how the Birmingham School Board approached the issue of mental disability and special education.

The proactive approach of Birmingham authorities in attempting to provide educational provision for those that were described as defective was not mirrored in all areas and the Mental Deficiency Act, 1913 in an attempt to impose some kind of uniformity, defined four classes of the mentally defective population. These were idiots, imbeciles, feeble-minded and the morally defective; the latter category was appropriated to include single unmarried mothers, demonstrating the fluid nature of definition and the moralistic concerns of authorities. Yet as Wynter has observed, the definitions of mental impairment fluctuated when deployed at the local level.[25] With local authorities, under the auspices of the newly formed Board of Control, given responsibility for the supervision and protection of defectives, both inside and outside of institutions it is important to assess how local ideas about mental capabilities formulated in practice.[26] This is possible for Birmingham thanks to a definitional exercise that took place two years prior to this seminal legislation. The Medical Superintendent of the Birmingham School Board, the Superintendent of Special Schools and the Chairman of the Special Schools Sub-Committee decided that clear classifications of mental deficiency in relation to the children already attending special classes in the city was required, in order to better understand the level of demand in Birmingham. This exercise created the local boundaries found in Table 4.2.

Unsurprisingly, children in Class V were the least ubiquitous in Birmingham's special schools while those in Class IV, those potentially requiring care into adulthood, were the most common. The description of each class was shaped around social and economic factors, rather than medical concerns. For instance, any child counted in Classes I through IV was only included because their families were judged not to have the means to assist them when they reached the age of 16, thus excluding them from Class V. In addition, Classes II and III were primarily linked to social efficiency and economic potential, whereas I and IV were concerned with the expense that might be incurred to the public purse. This echoes the findings of the Royal Commission on the Care and Control of the Feeble-Minded whose report in 1908 informed the

Table 4.2 Classification of the special school population in the Birmingham area, 1911

Class I	Cases urgently in need of further care and control; suitable for Residential Schools for the mentally defective
Class II	Cases that have a chance of becoming self-supporting
Class III	Cases that may become temporary wage-earners but that will need further care and control on the break-up of their homes
Class IV	Cases that will need further care and control in an institution at 16 or when they leave the Day Schools
Class V	Cases where parents will be in a position to look after them when they leave—well to do parents

Source Wolfson Centre for Archival Research, Special School Minute Book 1, BCC1/BH/5/1/1/1, p. 395

Mental Deficiency Act. Ellen Pinsent, the only female Commissioner and a key personality in driving the direction of educational provision in Birmingham, stated in 1909:

> There are numbers of mentally-defective persons whose training is neglected, over whom no sufficient control is exercised, and whose wayward and irresponsible lives are productive of crime and misery, of much injury and mischief to themselves and to others, and of much continuous expenditure.[27]

The report also reinforced two stereotypes about the feeble-minded: the first, being that the condition replicated itself from one generation to the next and the second, that the feeble-minded were more likely to engage in vice and criminality. The managers of the Sandwell Hall School readily bought into these tropes. Their initial prospectus stated: 'The history of the lives of mentally-defective people shows that if at liberty they materially increase the numbers of paupers, criminals, inebriates, and prostitutes, while the children to whom they too often give birth cannot fail to sink into the dependent class'.[28] It was argued that the children of these parents fell into two categories: the first were the criminal, vicious and immoral and the second were those living in 'bad homes'. For those in the latter category, the issue was not in the physical structure of the home, although many children lived in far from ideal abodes, but rather the occupants, with parents depicted as 'vicious', neglectful and 'cruel'.[29] Due to these circumstances, it was considered that mentally impaired children had 'no chance of becoming good citizens' without some kind of guidance in the form of education.[30]

Sandwell Hall School

The buildings used for the Sandwell Hall School, an Institution for the Care of Mentally Defective Children, belonged to the Earl of Dartmouth and from 1897 to 1905 the Lunacy Commissioners of Birmingham used them to house 200 lunatic patients on the site.[31] These were mainly 'quiet and dependable' convalescent patients from the Winson Green Asylum and they demonstrate the site's utility as a medical space, rather than an educational one immediately prior to its conversion. It was located in 30 acres and 'the land included in the holding is sufficient for exercise purposes and for the cultivation of vegetables for use in the Institution'.[32] The school was founded in 1908 and opened its doors to children the following year, with space for 80 boys and 70 girls. The Staff were resident and included a matron and teachers, with a Medical Officer visiting frequently. Unlike the Sandlebridge School in Cheshire, it did not intend to offer permanent care of the individuals that attended, although this element of provision was included in the original documentation.

Sandwell Hall School's guiding principles closely reflected the findings of the Royal Commission; the building itself had strong links with confining lunatic patients and the idea for it came from Rev. Harold Nelson Burden a colleague on the Royal Commission on the Feeble-Minded of the school's Honorary Secretary, Mrs. Ellen Pinsent. Upon his death in 1930, Burden was acclaimed as a 'pioneer in the research of problems connected with mental deficiency' and had worked in British India and East London before founding the National Institutions for Persons Requiring Care and Control.[33] The school was also managed and supervised by a Committee of Visitors made up of influential members of the local community. It included: G. H. Kenrick as Chairman—also Chair of the Birmingham Education Committee; David Davis Chairman of the Birmingham Asylums Committee; H. J. Sayer and A. J. Norton both former Chairmen of the Birmingham Board of Guardians; William Brown the Chair of the Aston Board of Guardians; Joseph Walter the Chairman of the King's Norton Board of Guardians; four members of the Birmingham Education Committee; and Dr. Violet Hill who was a member of the Special Schools After-Care Committee. Nominally, this organisation managed Sandwell Hall but from the outset, Burden made it clear that the school was 'financially under my own control and direction'.[34] The appointment of the Council was effective in tying the school to prominent figures across the city who had vested interests in providing suitable instruction to children and Pinsent was the key to ensuring that the new educational endeavour gained traction. She had served on the Royal Commission on the Feeble-Minded (1904–1908), was a Commissioner on the Board of Control from 1921 to 1932, but most significantly was elected to the Birmingham School Board's Special Schools Committee on 19 June 1900 and chaired it from 1901.[35] Less than a year later the School Board founded, upon her suggestion, an After-Care Sub-Committee to monitor individuals who were no longer under the supervision of special schools,[36] thus demonstrating her influence in directing special educational policy across the city.[37] Additionally, her influence and expertise in the management of mental deficiency were far-reaching, as attested to by Margaret MacDowall who wrote a treatise on the training of mentally defective children in 1919. In her introduction, she noted that following the Mental Deficiency Act, 1913, she retired to focus on the education of 'only a few children' as she 'could not work under the inspection of those who possibly might be unsympathetic'.[38] However, following an inspection from Pinsent in July 1916 MacDowall was reinvigorated into her work and accredits the inspiration for writing her volume to Pinsent. Subsequently, Pinsent's influence in the field is not to be underestimated.

As might be expected, the fate of Sandwell Hall, and the children associated with it, was closely intertwined with the figures of Burden and Pinsent and the experience of this institution reveals much about attitudes towards unhealthy young minds at this time. The promotional material for the school heralded the social role that it would fulfil and stated that 'children of feeble mental capacity are peculiarly liable to fall into sexual vices'.[39] It went on to note that those subject to violent tendencies 'are brought under control if the children are removed from home surroundings'.[40] These tropes about mentally deficient children held social weight and subsequently mainstream schools were deemed unsuitable because 'defective' children were considered to 'be incurable truants, and receive no benefit from instruction in Day Schools, on account of the irregularity of their attendance'.[41] As we have seen in Birmingham, the School Board was particularly aware of the presence of children requiring special education and attempted to provide appropriate education for them.

The management of the school adopted an approach that meant those taken would not become accustomed to a lifestyle that they were considered unlikely to maintain upon on the termination of their time at the school. They stated, in correspondence to the Board of Education, 'In view of the fact that they are never likely to have a high wage-earning capacity, the Managers are of the opinion that the provision made should be on economical lines'.[42] Such a statement was about making sure that the children under care knew their position in society but also may have prevented some applications from parents who could have viewed Sandwell Hall as a desirable alternative to workhouse accommodation.[43]

There was also an economic concern for local authorities who had to find extra money to fund residential education for children who could not attend 'ordinary' day schools. The Sandwell Hall council was told that 'the Local Education Authority (LEA) will only send children to it if the amount for each child does not exceed £27.10'.[44] In this instance, the LEA was in a position where it could dictate price, this concentrated the minds of managers who had to balance financial pressures that were associated with the residential nature of their educational offer. In an attempt to relieve economic concerns, Pinsent wrote to the Board of Education suggesting that they employed a head teacher with the salary of £40 per year with board and lodging. The proposed salary was significantly below those of class teachers working in day special schools in Birmingham. The LEA recommended that an 'uncertificated Assistant Mistress' should earn the salary of between £70 and £80 per annum, a substantial discrepancy with the head teacher salary at Sandwell Hall even with board and lodging taken into account.[45]

The Board of Education met with Burden and Pinsent to discuss the matter further. During this meeting, Pinsent stated that they had advertised for the post of Headmistress on the proposed terms but 'only one answered and she was quite impossible'.[46] To widen the net it was suggested 'that the rule may be relaxed and that they may be at liberty to appoint an uncertified teacher to the post'.[47] Here we see the quality of instruction was directly balanced against the financial health of the school, even though Mr. Tabor of the Board of Education reported that 'they [Pinsent and Burden] are certain that they will then be able to obtain a really competent person'.[48] The paradoxical nature of this statement did not seem to worry Burden or Pinsent as they attempted to get more by paying less. Pinsent used some of the professional capital that she had accrued serving on the Royal Commission and found an ally in Dr. Eichholz, the Board of Education's Inspector of Special Schools. Who commented that 'there is much force in Mrs. Pinsent's arguments. They are going to take the worst cases who will never repay in their careers a large educational outlay'.[49] Eichholz argued in favour of the proposal to appoint an uncertified teacher because he believed that LEAs would never agree to pay fees equivalent to those found in mainstream schools. However, support was not universal with Tabor commenting 'I should have thought that the additional cost of a certified teacher would be very small, and hardly appreciable in so large a general expenditure'[50]; and George Newman, the Chief Medical Officer, stating 'the Regulations [for Defective and Epileptic Schools] of 11th July 1904 are absolutely binding, the Board being given no discretionary power, we must, I fear, tell Mrs. Pinsent that we cannot waive the requirements of paragraph 6(a)'.[51]

Before the Board of Education had reached a decision, Pinsent attempted to raise the stakes and wrote a letter to Dr. Eichholz informing him that she had decided to appoint Frances Dipper as the school's first Headmistress. Dipper was aged 28 and Pinsent provided a glowing reference of her professional qualities. Listing her experience working in both an elementary school and special school in Birmingham, at the latter she had 'distinguished herself by the control she has gained over some of the most difficult among the scholars'.[52] This appointment forced the Board to make a decision on recognising an uncertified teacher. Pinsent though sought to mitigate this issue and informed the Board that Dipper 'was not able to go to college or to read for her certificate, owing to home claims, her mother being a widow and relying on her for help both pecuniary and domestic'.[53] Dipper was depicted as exemplary and respectable and she fulfilled the expected gender roles of Edwardian women. Commenting on Pinsent's reputation the Board agreed to approve Miss Dipper as Headmistress subject to approval from the Inspector, the sympathetic Dr. Eichholz.

With Dipper in place as Headmistress, the cost per child was set at £24 per annum, inclusive of clothing expenses. Furthermore, word of the school had also spread and the LEAs of Worcester, Rochford Hundred, Hereford, Berkshire and Chester had agreed to send children to the school, as had the Poor Law Guardians of Aston, Leicester and Wolverhampton. The Board of Education and the Local Government Board conducted inspection of the school's standards, with the Board of Control taking over some of these duties from 1914.

Sandwell Hall was one strand of provision for mentally defective children in Birmingham and operated in conjunction with the day special schools that were managed by the Birmingham School Board and after 1902 the LEA. When Dr. Eichholz inspected the Bristol Street Special School in 1908, he noted that 'the following children William B., William L., Joseph D., Annie R., and Jas B. are in capable of receiving benefit from day school instruction, and should not continue on the roll of this school. They are fit cases for permanent care'.[54] This report sparked a reaction from the Special Schools Sub-Committee to the wider school population in Birmingham and they stated on 13 May 1908 that 'there are at least 40 cases of the above description in the special schools under this Committee's control, needing permanent care and suitable for a boarding school'.[55] To deal with such a problem it was decided that 'in view of the fact that Sandwell Hall will probably be filled during the next three months' the Committee should make contact with Rev. Burden and reserve the necessary spaces.[56] This, of course, was mutually beneficial to parties and Ellen Pinsent with her oversight of Sandwell Hall and special education ensured that Birmingham was in prime position to filter appropriate children towards the school. By examining the experiences of some of these 'appropriate' children, it is possible to glean a better understanding of Sandwell Hall, ideas of healthy minds, and those who were responsible for education.

On 23 April 1909, there were 20 children admitted to the school, its largest intake since opening.[57] This was followed by a steady flow of children, such as Alice T. and Albert B. who both entered on 21 May 1909 with the fees covered by public funds and Rebecca S. who was admitted 1 June 1909 with her parents contributing 1/per week. Rebecca S. demonstrates that although there had been a move towards compulsory state-funded education, for children living with learning difficulties the normal funding streams did not always apply and parental contributions were sought. In another case, Douglas H. aged 9 had been truanting from the George West Day School for Mentally Defective Children in the city. In October 1909, his father appeared before the Appeals Committee of the LEA to account for his absence from school. It was recorded that 'the lad appeared to be beyond his father's control and declined to go with the Guide provided by the Committee'. Due to the difficulty of the boy's behaviour, it was decided that he was unsuitable for a day school and arrangements were made for him to be admitted to Sandwell Hall.[58] In this instance, the only details that are presented about the child in question are their challenging behaviour, again providing an insight into the range of needs that were accommodated at Sandwell Hall.

With the complexities associated with the needs of children, it is worth remembering that Sandwell Hall was not simply a dumping ground for those who were unable to function in society but rather, it was expected to maintain and provide a suitable standard of education for its pupils.[59] Therefore, when Dr. Eichholz inspected the premises in 1910, he found that four children, John W. (aged 14), Lily T. (14), Mary K. (12) and Annie R. (12), all previously removed from the Bristol Street School, were deemed to be 'uneducable' and should be removed from the roll. Despite their unsuitability, the Birmingham Special Schools Sub-Committee noted that 'in the event of these children leaving the institution arrangement be made where possible for them to be admitted to Day Schools in the City'.[60] This suggests that in this instance at least, the school space was used to control and supervise these children instead of being part of a concerted attempt to improve their educational and intellectual achievements. In a notable aside, John W.'s parents were chased for an outstanding contribution of 3/for his time in Sandwell Hall. Prosecution was discussed but it is uncertain if this action ever came to fruition.

It is evident from the classifications of children admitted to the school that there were tensions between central legislation and local practice. These tensions also manifested in the governance of the school and on the 13 October 1909 the Special School Sub-Committee at Birmingham was informed via its Chairman, Ellen Pinsent, of the resignation of the Sandwell Hall Council. It was resolved that Rev. Burden would be asked to furnish details of the new methods and conditions for governing the school and to provide 'full information' as to the new management committee.[61] Furthermore, Councillor Kenrick, previously the Chairman of the Sandwell Hall Council, and Councillor Jephcott, were appointed as LEA visitors for the school with responsibility for making sure it met local standards. This occurrence was a schism in the operation of the school. Only a month earlier, on 15 September 1909, a letter was submitted to the Special Schools Sub-Committee (chaired by Pinsent) from the Honorary Secretary of Sandwell Hall (also Pinsent), with regard to the opening of a new school at Stoke Park near Bristol, by the National Institutions for Persons Requiring Care and Control with Rev. Burden as the Warden. Rather than noting the impending implosion of Sandwell Hall, the committee decided to speak to the relevant Poor Law Guardians of the city with a view to admitting Amy T. and

Frank K. who had both been deemed too 'low grade' for education at Sandwell Hall.[62] Therefore, it appears that space to accommodate such children was at premium and the committee were willing to overlook the mismanagement of the school in order to find spaces for Birmingham children. Those children that were unsuitable for Sandwell Hall should have been maintained in an Idiot or Imbecile Asylum but space inside them was at a premium and private institutions required a nomination.[63]

Following the resignation of the council, and subsequent inadequate communication from Rev. Warden regarding the future direction of the school, it was resolved at the December meeting of the Special Schools Sub-Committee 'that no more children be sent to [Sandwell] Hall... until the Board of Education signify their approval of the new conditions under which the institution will be managed'.[64] It was not until April 1910 that such reassurance was given, even though it was accompanied, when it did arrive, by the caveat that approval was only a temporary measure for twelve months while they awaited a more secure plan for the management of the school. We thus see that the education of children considered to have unhealthy minds was at the whim of personal disputes and political decisions on both the local and national stage.

In 1911, a local examination of all children in Birmingham's special schools was carried out using the classification system discussed above in Table 4.2. The purpose was to identify the number of children requiring residential care and the likelihood of the special school population to be in some way self-supporting in adult life. Included in the survey were 837 children with the results displayed in Table 4.3.

Table 4.3 Birmingham Special School survey, 1911

	Boys	*Girls*	*Total*	*Percentage*
Class I—Residential schools	58	65	123	14.7
Class II—Chance of being self supporting	135	72	207	24.7
Class III—Temporary wage earners	141	74	215	25.7
Class IV—Further control post-16	152	128	280	33.5
Class V—Well to do families	8	4	12	1.4

Source Wolfson Centre for Archival Research, Special School Minute Book 1, BCC1/BH/5/1/1/1, p. 394

Alongside the broad classification, a more nuanced medical assessment of mentally defective children was also conducted. This found that there were 48 children in Birmingham suffering from epilepsy, but not mental deficiency and a further 23 in the extended city area. There were 9 children with combined epilepsy and mental deficiency, with 11 in the wider city area; and 111 mentally defective children without epilepsy and 52 in the wider city area.[65] Significantly, these counting exercises were designed not to ascertain the amount of room in Sandwell Hall that the Birmingham LEA required but rather as part of a plan to include mentally defectives in the Board's Monyhull Epileptic Colony, thus circumventing the reliance on Sandwell Hall. The Special Schools Sub-Committee concluded that the numbers had most likely been underestimated due to some parents not wanting to commit their children to specialist education until legislation compelled them to do so. Nevertheless they noted that 'during the next few years the Guardians would require places for 130 children and the Education Committee about 260 children, provision would be made for careful classification of the children, as the colony is to consist of detached homes'.[66] These comments signalled a shift in approach to directing children requiring residential care to the Monyhull Colony. The impact on Sandwell Hall was the loss of its most prolific contributor of children and subsequently a substantial reduction in revenue. In a further blow to Sandwell Hall, Ellen Pinsent and David Davies, formerly on the Council at the school, took up new roles on a committee to oversee the management of Monyhull, signalling a further distancing of the LEA from school.[67]

The financial consequences of the rift between the two parties were most starkly evidenced in the payments made by the LEA to the school. In October 1909, the Birmingham LEA paid the sum of £219 6s 8d for the maintenance of children present at Sandwell Hall. Three years later, in October 1912, the payment had reduced to £48 4s 10d for nine girls who the LEA had struggled to find alternative places for.[68] The school struggled on until 1921 but it was blighted by financial concerns and inability, in a time of expanding numbers of the mentally deficient, to fill its spaces. This was compounded by the reluctance of Rev. Burden to commit more of his own resources to the school and frequent requests from him to the Board of Education for an advance in grant payments that central government paid to special schools for each eligible pupil that was present. In 1921, the situation at the school had deteriorated to such an extent that the Board of Education refused to recertify the school citing 'serious irregularities'.[69] Burden attempted to appeal, stating 'the defects in the school, such as they are, are wholly traceable to the lack of funds due to the exceedingly small amount paid for maintenance'.[70] The Board did not reconsider and the Sandwell Hall School subsequently closed in December 1921, with its buildings demolished seven years later.

Conclusions

The experience of the Sandwell Hall School reveals that efforts at caring for and managing the healthy minds of children at the beginning of the twentieth century were centred on the intellectual and moral health of the child. Operating in a compulsory and state education system it was inevitable that ideas of mental deficiency were influenced by national and local inputs. Sandwell Hall grew out of wider concerns, its founders meeting as they worked on the Royal Commission on the Feeble-Minded together, work that they both considered essential to the national interest. The focus of Burden and Pinsent was on attempting to ameliorate the mental conditions of children and the school was founded on a belief that education would materially benefit the individual, both immediately and in their later life. However, in practice, interventions were symbolic of power struggles that existed about how best to manage this specific population of children in order to educate them into a socially efficient, 'healthy' and independent-minded members of the population. In the end, the Sandwell Hall School descended into farce and economic ruin, with the interests of its pupils and their 'unhealthy' minds apparently secondary to personal ambitions.

Acknowledgements This research was completed as part of my Wellcome Trust Institutional Strategic Support Fellowship Early Career Award held at the University of Leicester, 204801/Z/16/Z.

Notes

1. Matthew Thomson, *Psychological Subjects: Identity, Culture, and Health in Twentieth-Century Britain* (Oxford: Oxford University Press, 2006), 111.
2. Mark Jackson, *The Borderland of Imbecility: Medicine, Society and the Fabrication of the Feeble Mind in Late Victorian and Edwardian England* (Manchester: Manchester University Press, 2000).

3. Mark Jackson, "Institutional Provision for the Feeble-Minded in Edwardian England: Sandlebridge and the Scientific Morality of Permanent Care," in *From Idiocy to Mental Deficiency: Historical Perspectives on People with Learning Disabilities*, eds. A. Digby and D. Wright (London: Routledge, 1996), 161–183.
4. David Daniel, "The Ineducable Children of Leeds: The Operation of the Defective Children and Mental Deficiency Legislation in Leeds, 1900–29," *Journal of Educational Administration and History* 29, no. 2 (July 1997): 121–141, 122.
5. Daniel, "The Ineducable Children of Leeds," 123.
6. Pamela Dale, "Special Education at Starcross Before 1948," *History of Education* 36, no. 1 (2007): 17–44, 20.
7. Rebecca Wynter, "Pictures of Peter Pan: Institutions, Local Definitions of 'Mental Deficiency,' and the Filtering of Children in Early Twentieth-Century England," *Family and Community History* 18, no. 2 (November 2015): 122–138.
8. Michel Foucault, *Madness and Civilization: A History of Insanity in the Age of Reason* (London: Routledge, reprinted 2001), originally published as *Histoire de la Folie* (Paris: Plon, 1964); Andrew Scull, *Museums of Madness: The Social Organization of Insanity in Nineteenth-Century England* (London: Allen Lane, 1979); Peter Bartlett, *The Poor Law of Lunacy: The Administration of Pauper Lunatics in Mid-Nineteenth-Century England* (London: Leicester University Press, 1999); Joseph Melling and Bill Forsythe, eds., *Insanity, Institutions, and Society, 1800–1914: A Social History of Madness in Comparative Perspective* (London: Routledge, 1999).
9. David Wright, *Mental Disability in Victorian England: The Earlswood Asylum, 1847–1901* (Oxford: Clarendon, 2001); Amy Rebok-Rosenthal, "Insanity, Family and Community in Late-Victorian Britain," in *Disabled Children Contested Caring, 1850–1979*, eds. A. Borsay and P. Dale (London: Pickering and Chatto, 2012), 29–42; Steven J. Taylor, *Child Insanity in England, 1845–1907* (Basingstoke: Palgrave Macmillan, 2017); Steven J. Taylor, "'She Was Frightened While Pregnant by a Monkey at the Zoo': Constructing the Mentally-Imperfect Child in Nineteenth-Century England," *Social History of Medicine* 30, no. 4 (November 2017): 748–766.
10. *British Library Newspapers*, "Care of the Feeble-Minded." Cambridge Independent Press, 12 March 1909, 7. http://link.galegroup.com/apps/doc/JF3240702317/DSLAB?u=leicester&sid=DSLAB&xid=dafcba9f. Accessed 1 April 2019.
11. Taylor, *Child Insanity in England.*
12. See Taylor, *Child Insanity in England*, Introduction.

13. G. Newman, *Infant Mortality: A Social Problem* (London: Methuen, 1906), 7.
14. G. E. Shuttleworth, *Mentally Deficient Children: Their Treatment and Training* (London: H.K. Lewis, 1895), Preface.
15. See Taylor, *Child Insanity in England*, for a more comprehensive discussion of definitions.
16. Shuttleworth, *Mentally Deficient Children*, for more information on educational, see 72; industrial 90, and moral 96.
17. Shuttleworth, *Mentally Deficient Children*, 90.
18. Ibid., 92.
19. Jackson, *Borderland of Imbecility*.
20. Shuttleworth, *Mentally Deficient Children*, 97–98.
21. A. Binet and T. Simon, *Mentally Defective Children* (London: Edward Arnold, 1914).
22. Binet and Simon, *Mentally Defective Children*, 10.
23. Wolfson Centre for Archival Research (Henceforth WCAR) SB/B11/1/1/1, Birmingham Education Committee, Special Schools Committee of the School Board Minutes, 10 February 1898–17 March 1903, 111.
24. WCAR, SB/B11/1/1/1, Special Schools Committee of the School Board Minutes, 10 February 1898–17 March 1903, 214.
25. Wynter, "Pictures of Peter Pan."
26. Pamela Dale, "Implementing the 1913 Mental Deficiency Act," *Social History of Medicine* 16, no. 3 (December 2003): 403–418.
27. "Care of the Feeble-Minded." http://link.galegroup.com/apps/doc/JF3240702317/DSLAB?u=leicester&sid=DSLAB&xid=dafcba9f. Accessed 1 April 2019.
28. The National Archives (Henceforth TNA), ED32/187, Sandwell Hall Prospectus.
29. Ibid.
30. Ibid.
31. TNA, ED32/187, Letter from Rev. Burden, 22 September 1906.
32. TNA, ED32/187, Sandwell Hall Prospectus.
33. The Times Digital Archive (Henceforth TDA), *The Times*, "The Rev. H. N. Burden," 29 May 1930, 18. http://link.galegroup.com/apps/doc/CS302981821/DSLAB?u=leicester&sid=DSLAB&xid=25ab4767. Accessed 1 April 2019.
34. TNA, Sandwell Hall Application to the Board of Education for Certificate, ED32/187.
35. TDA, *The Times*, "Dame Ellen Pinsent," 21 October 1949, 7. http://link.galegroup.com/apps/doc/CS120277333/DSLAB?u=leicester&sid=DSLAB&xid=cee2dde0. Accessed 1 April 2019.

36. WCAR, SB/B11/1/1/1, Special Schools Committee of the School Board Minutes, 10 February 1898–17 March 1903, 96 and 127.
37. Ibid.
38. M. MacDowall, *Simple Beginnings in the Training of Mentally Defective Children* (London: Local Government Press, 1919), Introduction.
39. TNA, ED32/187, Sandwell Hall Prospectus.
40. Ibid.
41. Ibid.
42. Ibid.
43. For examples, see Cathy Smith, "Family, Community and the Victorian Asylum: A Case Study of the Northampton General Lunatic Asylum and Its Pauper Lunatics," *Family and Community History* 9, no. 2 (November 2006): 109–124.
44. TNA, ED32/187, Copy of Memorandum of Interview Between Mrs. Pinsent, Rev. H. N. Burden and Mr. Tabor, 4 February 1907.
45. WCAR, SB/B11/1/1/1, Special Schools Committee of the School Board Minutes, 10 February 1898–17 March 1903, 218.
46. TNA, ED32/187, Copy of Memorandum of Interview Between Mrs. Pinsent, Rev. H. N. Burden, and Mr. Tabor, 4 February 1907.
47. Ibid.
48. Ibid.
49. Ibid.
50. Ibid.
51. Ibid.
52. TNA, ED32/187, Letter from Mrs. Pinsent to the Board of Education, 19 March 1907.
53. Ibid.
54. WCAR, BCC1/BH/5/1/1/2, Special School Minute Book 2, 414.
55. Ibid.
56. Ibid.
57. Ibid., 333.
58. WCAR, BCC1/BH/5/1/1/1, Special School Minute Book 1, 122.
59. A similar argument for pauper lunatic asylums in the nineteenth century, see Andrew Scull, *Museums of Madness: The Social Organization of Insanity in Nineteenth-Century England* (London: Allen Lane, 1979).
60. WCAR, BCC1/BH/5/1/1/1, Special School Minute Book 1, 280.
61. Ibid., 122.
62. Ibid., 105.
63. Wright, *Mental Disability in Victorian England*.
64. WCAR, BCC1/BH/5/1/1/1, Special School Minute Book 1, 141.
65. Ibid., 395.
66. Ibid.

67. Ibid.
68. WCAR, BCC1/BH/5/1/1/3, Special School Minute Book 3, 174.
69. TNA, ED32/187, Letter from the Board of Education to Rev. H. N. Burden, 27 May 1921.
70. TNA, ED32/187, Letter from Rev. H. N. Burden to the Board of Education, 30 June 1921.

CHAPTER 5

Healthy Minds and Intellectual Disability

Jan Walmsley

Introduction

This chapter concerns itself with the concept of a healthy mind as applied to people with intellectual or learning disabilities. It traces its roots back to the early part of the twentieth century, particularly the pervasive belief in eugenics, and uses historical practice and experience as a prism to consider the situation in the present. The principal argument is that people with intellectual or learning disabilities, by definition, do not have minds that can be regarded as 'healthy'. This is an important, if not controversial, starting point. If people with learning disabilities in the twenty-first century are to gain equal status as fellow citizens, as was promised in the Valuing People White Paper (England and Wales 2001), Same as You (Scotland 2000), and the United Nations Convention on the Rights of People with Disabilities to which the UK was a signatory in 2007 there needs to be a change that goes beyond stirring policy statements, a pious belief that things will get better, or even 'more resources'.[1] This chapter addresses two major questions; firstly, how far were people with intellectual disabilities regarded as having healthy minds during the twentieth century? And, secondly, what relevance does this have to people with learning or intellectual disabilities in the present?

J. Walmsley (✉)
Open University, Milton Keynes, UK

S. J. Taylor and A. Brumby (eds.), *Healthy Minds in the Twentieth Century*, Mental Health in Historical Perspective,
https://doi.org/10.1007/978-3-030-27275-3_5

This chapter will focus on a number of issues, including Western philosophy, eugenic theory, changing labels, psychotherapy and control of reproduction, in order to find answers to these questions.

Labels—Language and Its Significance

A brief discussion of language, especially the changing nature of labels applied to people currently known as having 'learning' or 'intellectual' disabilities, is essential to frame the analysis of the chapter. Alfred Tredgold, a highly influential doctor and member of the 1908 Radnor Commission, used the term 'amentia' (absence of mind) in early editions of his book *Mental Deficiency* which was the key textbook in medicine and nursing until the late twentieth century.[2] If the mind is associated with reason, perception, judgement, intellect and understanding, what does it mean not to have a mind, or to have a mind that is impaired? The early twentieth-century term 'feeble-minded' was officially adopted in legislation passed in 1913 in England and Wales and was widely used in the USA, Canada and the rest of the English-speaking world[3] although Steven Taylor observes in Chapter 4 of this volume that definitions could fluctuate according to space and place. The very use of the word 'feeble' means that these could not be considered healthy minds. 'Feeble-minded' was used as a social and medical category until the second half of the twentieth century, as the legislation which perpetuated it, the Mental Deficiency Act, 1913, was not repealed until 1959. Indeed, 'feeble-minded' lingered on in common speech beyond that time. A parent in an interview used it with the author in 1991 to describe another parent who had two children with learning disabilities.[4] The word 'ineducable' was introduced into official language in 1944, to label those deemed incapable of benefitting from an education also suggests that medically and legally a mind was considered less than healthy if it was incapable of education. These children were only admitted to the education system in 1970.

The Mental Deficiency Act, 1913 subdivided the term 'defectives', into the following classifications: 'idiots', 'imbeciles', 'feeble minded' and 'moral defectives'. These were replaced in the Mental Health Act, 1959, by the terminology 'sub-normal', which was then itself replaced by 'mental handicap', 'learning disabilities', and now the term 'intellectual disabilities' appears to be gaining favour. Alongside these legal and medical classifications, have been less formal designations like 'backward', applied to children until well into the late twentieth century, and also terms which started life as having a medical significance, like 'mongol' and 'cretin' but which quickly degenerated into terms of abuse. In the final quarter of the twentieth century, there was a shift towards the language of disability/disabled. This realignment, from association with madness and mental affliction to association with people who are physically impaired has been significant—for example, it opened the way for the influence of the social model of disability to learning disability.[5] The shift has, in some respects, left people marooned between the two and neglected by both.[6] Paradoxically, the medical specialty most closely associated with learning/intellectual disability remains psychiatry, despite the official dropping of the 'mental' label. The connection with 'learning' remains in 'learning disabled' and its user preferred variant 'learning difficulties'. In the internationally used variant 'intellectual disabilities', the problem remains in the mind, specifically with the intellect.

Valerie Sinason, leading psychotherapist, is of the view that the ever-changing labels, and the bitter conversations accompanying debates about the proper language to use, are no coincidence. They are a means to hide deep discomfort about 'learning disability' as a toxic identity, the ultimate outgroup.[7] In a world where intellect, reason and judgement are paramount marks of esteem, to be labelled as lacking these, is indeed stigmatising. Despite the shift to apparently less stigmatising language—intellectual disability is preferable to 'feeble-minded' or 'idiot' to the modern ear—the abbreviation ID for 'intellectual disability' is widely used in academic papers. It seems somewhat disrespectful, distancing and dehumanising to abbreviate what is supposed to be a respectful modern term, but it is a common practice.

The Eugenic Influence and Legacy

The spectre of eugenics cannot be separated from terms such as defective, idiot, imbecile and feeble-minded. It would have come as a surprise to campaigners and legislators of the early twentieth century to find the idea of healthy minds applied to what were then generically called 'mental defectives'. The minds of these people were, according to the official Radnor Report (1908), so diseased as to be 'a terrible danger to the race' (a phrase attributed to Winston Churchill).[8] At the turn of the nineteenth and twentieth centuries, Binet's IQ tests were deployed to show that most convicts and prostitutes were illiterate and therefore feeble-minded.[9] These tests provided quasi-scientific truths that these people were the cause of many of the ills with which society grappled—illegitimacy, drunkenness, promiscuity and fecklessness to name but a few. So hideous was this often hidden danger—the feeble-minded could often pass as normal—that they needed to be sought out, ascertained and detained in segregated institutions.[10] There was a belief that feeble-mindedness was hereditary and unless the breeding of the feeble-minded was curtailed, the 'healthy' stock would, it was believed, be overwhelmed by larger numbers of defectives. US Scientist H. H. Goddard affirmed that feeble-minded people were 'multiplying at twice the rate of the general population',[11] thus producing 'more feeble-minded children with which to clog the wheels of human progress'.[12] He too cited quasi-scientific research to back up these claims. Goddard met a young woman whom he called Deborah Kallikak in an institution and later looked into her family tree. Her great-grandfather had been Martin Kallikak. According to Goddard, the Kallikak family was divided into two strains—one 'good' and one 'bad'—both of which originated from Martin Kallikak, Sr. The 'Normal N' and 'Feeble Minded F' were deduced by what these ancestors achieved in their lives. When Martin Kallikak, Sr. was a young soldier, he had a liaison with an 'unnamed, feeble-minded tavern girl'. This relationship resulted in the birth of an illegitimate son, Martin Kallikak, Jr. It was argued that the 'bad' strain of the Kallikak family descended from this line. Later Martin Kallikak, Sr., married a Quaker woman from a 'good' family. The 'good' line descended from this marriage. Goddard's genealogical research purported to show that the union with the feeble-minded tavern girl resulted in generations of 'mental defectives' who were plagued by illegitimacy, prostitution, alcoholism, epilepsy and lechery. His investigation into the other Kallikak branch revealed the opposite: Goddard believed that the striking schism separating the two branches of the family was due entirely to the different genetic input from the women.[13]

In the UK, the Mental Deficiency Act 1913 was introduced in direct response to the moral panic associated with these eugenic beliefs. This legislation made it possible to segregate 'defectives' in institutions, with men and women kept strictly apart to prevent 'breeding'.[14] Other measures to restrict childbearing, associated with negative eugenics, included prohibition of marriage, which was widely canvassed in England during the 1920s, legalised sterilisation, and other forms of birth control.[15] None of these were formally adopted in any of the British Isles, but sterilisation was widely practised.[16]

The heyday of segregation as the preferred way to manage mental defectives, and to prevent their breeding, was the first three-quarters of the twentieth century. In the Western world at least, following scandals and journalistic exposes, buildings based on the idea of segregation in large remote 'colonies' fell out of fashion.[17] However, these buildings and institutions continue to be the dominant form of provision, other than family-based care, in much of the rest of the world.

In the countries of the west, which had been amongst the earliest to adopt a 'colony' solution, a combination of factors came together to bring that era to an end. Segregation was an expensive way to prevent the 'unfit' from having children once the employment of 'high grade' patients became unacceptable during the 1950s. At a time of high employment and rising wages, it became ever more difficult to recruit staff to work in remote institutions often run on quasi-military lines.[18] Academic critiques, such as that of Goffman[19] and parent-run organisations like the National Association of Parents of Backward Children (England), and the National Association for Retarded Children (USA) also exerted pressure on politicians to move cautiously away from institutional solutions.[20] The last large state-run institutions to open in the UK were in the early 1970s at Princess Marina Hospital in Northampton, and Lea Castle Hospital in Kidderminster: the last one to officially close was Orchard Hill, on the outskirts of London in 2010. However, the demise of the institutional solution did not signal a true reappraisal of people with learning disabilities, rather it proved that technology opened the way for new forms of reproductive control, negating the need for physical segregation.

Sterilisation and Contraception

Control of reproduction was the driving force behind segregationist policies. The arrival of more effective contraception meant that physical segregation became less necessary. Sterilisation also offered an alternative to achieving the pre-eminent eugenic aim of preventing procreation and child-rearing by people with feeble-minds. In numerous countries, including many states of the USA, Canada, Sweden and Iceland, involuntary sterilisation was practised lawfully during much of the twentieth century.[21] In Sweden, Iceland and the USA, it was a condition of release from the institution.[22] Oral history accounts provide a greater degree of insight, such as this recollection from Ragnheiður, a former inmate of an Icelandic institution:

> It is so strange. When I moved to the group home I had to undergo sterilization. I didn't agree but I had to agree because otherwise I would not be allowed to move from the institution.[23]

Sociologist Robert Edgerton, writing in the 1960s, noted that 44 of the 48 ex-patients he interviewed about life outside had been subject to 'eugenic sterilisation' before their release from the Pacific State Colony, California.[24] The letter sent from the Colony seeking parental permission emphasised that it would enable parole and visits outside, and unless there were strong objections, the patient was sterilised. Edgerton records that a few respondents, all single men, approved of the operation, giving them greater freedom. However, most regretted it, and several saw it as a 'permanent source of doubt about their mental state'.[25] One woman speculated a connection with an unhealthy mind in her musing to the researcher on the subject:

> I still don't know why they did that surgery to me. The sterilization wasn't for punishment, was it? Was it because there was something wrong with my mind?[26]

Edgerton noted that the most significant cause of concern was the difficulty it posed for hiding a discredited past, to tell or not to tell potential partners—or in the terms of this volume, to conceal the diagnosis of not having an acceptably healthy mind. The resulting scar was regularly explained as the result of an appendectomy. Edgerton notes the irony that this was how the hospital explained the operation, saying to patients that it was to remove an appendix, a subterfuge that was also recorded in England, Canada and Iceland.[27]

Famously, in the four countries of the UK involuntary sterilisation was never legalised after the failure of the Brock Committee to persuade Parliament to legislate in the 1930s.[28] Nevertheless, this did not mean it did not occur as shown by Tilley et al. via oral histories, and by Stansfield et al. who scrutinised court records of the later twentieth century.[29] Sterilisation was widely canvassed in the mid- and later twentieth century. A survey undertaken in England in the 1990s found that over half of 274 responding family members would or had considered sterilisation for their child.[30] Roy et al.'s study found that family members considering sterilisation had not explored alternative contraception.[31] In 2011, the author interviewed two elderly parents of a woman born in 1950 who recounted how they had obtained sterilisation for their daughter in 1970 by requesting it from the GP.[32] Their fear was, not that she would have sex, which she apparently much enjoyed, but that it would result in a child that she would be unable to adequately care for. Ladd-Taylor argues that it was child-rearing that was the focus, not childbearing:

> Sterilization policy was as much about preventing child rearing by the so-called feeble minded as it was about preventing child bearing.[33]

The most recent study on the subject of sterilisation in England and Wales was a detailed review of 73 applications which went before the Official Solicitor between 1988 and 1999.[34] Seventy of these cases were women, three were men, and 37% were minors. The average age of the women was 21.4 years. The court approved thirty-one sterilisations; six procedures went ahead without the need for court approval because it was deemed 'therapeutic'. Thus, roughly half the cases that were considered were deemed suitable for sterilisation.

There is little evidence about sterilisation practices after this period, despite the implementation of the Mental Capacity Act 2005, in England and Wales, which arguably provided a new framework for decision-making in relation to reproductive rights. However, evidence about recent practice from other countries shows that sterilisation remains widespread. A Belgian study of 397 women aged 18–46 found that 22% had been sterilised.[35] A Dutch study involving 397 women aged 15–59 of whom 112 were using contraception, found that 25 had been sterilised, 20 of these prior to 2000.[36] Intellectually disabled people may be sterilised, without their consent, under New Zealand law, and court authorisation is not always necessary.[37] Concern about people with intellectual or learning disabilities reproducing continues in twenty-first-century thinking and practice. It is estimated that between 40 and 60% of children born to parents with intellectual disabilities in Western countries are removed from their care.[38]

The drive to prevent people with 'unhealthy' minds from having children has not ended, but it is much less visible and in the UK sterilisation appears to no longer be widely practised. The literature indicates that in the early twenty-first century, women's capacity to conceive and bear children is, in the main, controlled through social and contraceptive care interventions rather than surgical sterilisation.[39] While the law in England and Wales has changed to make sterilisation without legal sanction virtually impossible, 'newgenic' social practices continue to restrict the sexual and reproductive freedoms of learning disabled women. Tilley et al. comment:

> Whilst medical technologies may have changed, essential questions about intellectually disabled women's rights to participate in decisions about their own reproductive futures remain.[40]

McCarthy and Ledger et al. argue that continuing use of long-acting patches to prevent pregnancy is a form of reproductive control which does not require legal sanction.[41] Two small-scale studies indicated that many women with intellectual disabilities are prescribed long-acting contraception without requesting it, frequently when they are not in relationships.[42]

This discussion of reproductive control concludes with an exploration of policy changes. Policy statements of the twenty-first century are bold, optimistic and unambiguous, for instance England's *Valuing People Now* explicitly stated, 'people with learning disabilities have the choice to have relationships, become parents and continue to be parents and are supported to do so'.[43] Yet the gap between rhetoric and reality is yawning. Prevention of childbearing and child-rearing continues to inform practice, under a cloak of changing policy. The drive to privilege reproduction of 'healthy minds', untainted by intellectual disability, has not gone away.

Normalisation and Social Role Valorisation

Normalisation and social role valorisation are perhaps the most explicit acknowledgement in theory that it matters to hide the unhealthy mind. The question of how to address what appeared to be the low valuation of people with intellectual disabilities became a preoccupation of the late twentieth century. Drawing on sociologist Goffman's argument that to overcome stigma, it was essential to 'pass' as normal, to conceal the discrediting attributes, normalisation and social role valorisation, came to dominate learning disability policy and practice from the 1970s onwards.[44] Normalisation was defined by Dane Bank Mikkelson as letting the mentally handicapped (sic) obtain an existence as close to normal as possible.[45] These ideas from the Nordic countries were recast by, the American theorist, Wolf Wolfensberger as social role valorisation:

> The utilization of means which are as culturally normative as possible in order to establish and / or maintain personal behaviours which are as culturally normative as possible.[46]

To achieve this, a positive image of people with learning disabilities was vital as it would assist in people being accepted in mainstream society. Social role valorisation emphasised the importance of people with learning disabilities taking on 'valued social roles'—if people with learning disabilities occupied valued roles such as worker—or researcher—then fuller integration into society would become possible. Wolfensberger also advocated association with 'valued', i.e. non-disabled people. It was, I would suggest, a way of concealing their stigma of an 'unhealthy' mind, as the route to wider acceptance.

Eradication

The final example of the 'low' value which has historically been attributed to people with learning disabilities is their potential for eradication. This practice was associated with the Nazis in the mid-twentieth century when they murdered people that they labelled Unnütze Esser or, in English, 'useless eaters'.[47] It was, until quite recently, believed that this had discredited eugenics, and that the eradication of people with learning disabilities is no longer countenanced.[48] Wolf Wolfensberger, mentioned above as the architect of social role valorisation, disagreed. His view was that 'deathmaking' is one of the functions of learning disability services. He cited case studies which demonstrated how medical services fail disabled people, primarily because to some their lives are still perceived to have low quality and value.[49] He wrote:

> handicapped people are given massive doses of psychoactive drugs so that they die from drug effects – even though the death certificate will list only the complications such as cardiac arrest, pneumonia.[50]

Within his work, he also targeted abortion. He drew parallels between Nazi Germany's extermination practices and contemporary practice of aborting disabled foetuses.[51]

> I think that the liberalisation of abortion is one of the expressions of the lowering of human life and I do believe we will soon see legalised euthanasia. We will see it applied to the aged and the retarded first .... We will

> have to see that you can't have this part way; that once you break through a qualitative barrier of defining human life and its value, then there's no stopping.[52]

Some recent events suggest that Wolfensberger's views cannot be lightly dismissed. The poor health care offered to people with learning disabilities revealed in Mencap's *Death by Indifference* campaign and the findings of the University of Bristol's Confidential Enquiry into Premature Death (CIPOLD) can both be considered to be evidence of this.[53] Moreover, the failure to investigate unexpected and premature deaths to which the Mazars Report drew attention, reinforced by the Care Quality Commission's findings in 2016, is further evidence to point to the low value which, in some contexts, continues to be accorded to the lives of people with learning disabilities.[54]

Wolfensberger's starting point for arguing that we are on a slippery slope to discarding lives perceived by others to be of 'low value' was the widespread practice of aborting foetuses identified as disabled through prenatal testing.[55] Recent medical 'advances' open up the real possibility that Down's Syndrome will be eradicated entirely by early detection in utero, followed by abortion, discussed in Sally Phillips's TV Programme *A World Without Down Syndrome* first broadcast in 2016.[56] Genetics offers the potential to identify more traits than Down's Syndrome in utero which as long ago as 1977 Reilly cited as having the potential for negative eugenics.[57] If the gene for autism can be located, for example, it opens the way for this also to be detected and eradicated before birth. Barnbaum uses absence of theory of mind to argue that parents have a moral obligation not to bring autistic individuals into the world, although she argues that once born, a different approach needs to prevail.[58] It is difficult to escape the view that the emphasis on 'healthy minds' in modern discourse continues to influence policy and practice in relation to the abortion of disabled foetuses.

Despite this discussion, the question remains why, despite modern policies and stirring words, do people with learning disabilities continue, in certain contexts, to have such low social value and how might this be rectified? This returns us right back to the idea of 'healthy minds' as a concept. In 2008, before things got as bad as they were at the time of writing (see, for example, the UN's condemnation of UK's failure to uphold the CPRD 2016),[59] Kelley Johnson and I pondered the question—why, after 3 decades of social inclusion policies, a good life for people with learning disabilities seemed so elusive.[60] We looked at Western philosophy for answers. We found that 'reason' was pre-eminent in the qualities philosophers valued for a rounded life. Overwhelmingly, male philosophers have outlawed emotions and passion as disturbing to the equilibrium sought through the exercise of reason. Of particular significance was the view associated with the eighteenth-century Enlightenment which equated human history with progress related to man's reason, increasing knowledge and understanding of the natural world, and the means to control it. Certainly, the implications of not being seen to possess reason run deep. John Rawls argued that as rational human beings we develop a social contract resting on two principles. The first is the freedom to pursue the life we want to lead providing it does not harm others. The second is that economic and social inequality is unavoidable, but the institutions of society should protect the less well off.[61] Like many preceding philosophers—John Locke amongst them—Rawls assumed that a social contract existed between individuals who are equal to one another in their freedom to suggest how society should be organised, based on their reasoning and ability to participate. People with learning disabilities are those whose interests must be protected in a Rawlsian sense, rather than being active citizens who participate in formulating a just and fair society. There is a fundamental inequality here, built into the social contract.

Notoriously, twentieth-century thinker Peter Singer placed reason at the core of what makes us human and used this to exclude many people with learning disabilities from the status of human being.[62] This extolling of reason, we argued then, is at the core of the exclusion of people with learning disabilities. Subsequently, another advocate for people with learning disabilities, Chris Goodey argued that since the eighteenth-century Enlightenment, if not before, people now called learning disabled have been the ultimate outgroup.[63] He traces this to the pre-eminence of intellectual ability in modern claims to species membership; he stated that 'intellectual ability or intelligence is in modern societies the foremost claim to status'.[64] This, he argued, is used to justify classifying people with learning disabilities as an outgroup, suggesting that 'classifying a human group by intellectual criteria is today's prevailing symptom of inclusion phobia'.[65] He further develops the argument to say that 'intellectual disability is vital to the dominant in-group because of its relationship to that quality which that group attributes to itself'.[66] In other words, we need people with learning disabilities to prove our intellectual ability—there is no point in having it—if everyone has it. Unless this idea changes, he argues, no amount of bold pronouncements will produce change. Taken together, these two attempts at understanding the persistent othering of people with intellectual disabilities alluded to in this chapter are depressing. However, unless these conclusions are faced up to and challenged for what they are, change will only be superficial, and only for the few who can—as numerous self-advocates assert—do things other people can do.

Conclusions

This chapter has argued that some of the impulses that drove the movement to privilege and protect 'healthy minds', by segregating people with intellectual disabilities to prevent their 'breeding', have not vanished, as some would argue. Rather the desire to prevent childbearing and child-rearing remains, but thanks to technology, the means of prevention are far less obvious; they are well hidden under rhetorical flourishes proclaiming rights. Efforts to change this state of affairs, such as normalisation/social role valorisation, rely, not on challenging the fundamental undervaluing of people with intellectual disabilities, but on persuading people to 'pass' as normal, and persuading others to support such passing by offering and talking up 'valued social roles'. My challenge to readers is to recognise that until the overinflated value attributed to intellect and reason changes, until we re-evaluate what constitutes a 'healthy mind', such undervaluing will continue.

Notes

1. United Nations Convention on the Rights of Persons with Disabilities, *Inquiry Concerning the United Kingdom of Great Britain and Northern Ireland Carried Out by the Committee Under Article 6 of the Optional Protocol to the Convention: Report of the Committee* (Geneva: United Nations, 2016). www.ohchr.org/EN/HRBodies/CRPD/Pages/InquiryProcedure.aspx. Accessed 21 February 2017.
2. Alfred Tredgold, *Mental Deficiency: Amentia* (London: Baillière, Tindall and Cox, 1908); Michael Craft, *Tredgold's Mental Retardation* (12th edition) (Baillière, Tindall and Cox, 1979).
3. James W. Trent, *Inventing the Feeble Mind: A History of Mental Retardation in the United States* (Berkeley: California University Press, 1994).

4. Jan Walmsley, *Gender, Caring and Learning Disability* (Unpublished PhD thesis, The Open University, Milton Keynes, 1995).
5. Jan Walmsley, "Normalisation, Emancipatory Research and Learning Disability," *Disability and Society* 16, no. 2 (2001): 187–205.
6. Jane Campbell and Mike Oliver, *Disability Politics: Understanding Our Past, Changing Our Future* (London: Routledge, 1996).
7. See for instance, Valerie Sinason, *Mental Handicap and the Human Condition: New Approaches from the Tavistock* (London: Free Association Books, 1992); Christopher Goodey, *Learning Disability and Inclusion Phobia: Past, Present and Future* (London: Routledge, 2015); Stuart Todd and Julia Shearn "Family Dilemmas and Secrets: Parents' Disclosure of Information to Their Adults Offspring with Learning Disabilities," *Disability and Society* 12, no. 3 (1997): 341–366.
8. T. Stainton, "Equal Citizens? The Discourse of Liberty and Rights in the History of Learning Disabilities," in *Crossing Boundaries: Change and Continuity in the History of Learning Disability*, eds. L. Brigham D. Atkinson, M. Jackson et al. (Kidderminster: British Institute of Learning Disabilities, 2000), 87–102.
9. Craft, *Tredgold's Mental Retardation*, 5.
10. Jan Walmsley, Dorothy Atkinson, and Sheena Rolph, "Community Care and Mental Deficiency 1913–1945," in *Outside the Walls of the Asylum*, eds. Peter Bartlett and David Wright (London: The Athlone Press, 1999), 181–203; Mark Jackson, *The Borderland of Imbecility: Medicine, Society and the Fabrication of the Feeble Mind in Late Victorian and Edwardian England* (Manchester: Manchester University Press, 2000).
11. H. H. Goddard, *The Kallikak Family: A Study in the Heredity of Feeble-Mindedness* (New York: Macmillan, 1912), 71.
12. Ibid., 78.
13. Ibid., 105–106.
14. Greta Jones, *Social Hygiene in Twentieth Century Britain* (Worcester: Billing and Sons, 1986).
15. Dorothy Atkinson and Fiona Williams, eds. *Know Me as I Am* (London: Hodder and Stoughton, 1990); Walmsley, Atkinson, and Rolph, "Community Care."
16. Elizabeth Tilley, Jan Walmsley, Sarah Earle, and Dorothy Atkinson, "'The Silence Is Roaring': Sterilization, Reproductive Rights and Women with Intellectual Disabilities," *Disability and Society* 27, no. 3 (May 2012): 413–426.
17. John Welshman, "Organisations, Structures and Community Care 1948–71: From Control to Care," in *Community Care in Perspective,* eds. John Welshman and Jan Walmsley (London: Macmillan, 2006), 59–76.

18. Jan Walmsley, "Institutionalisation: An Historical Perspective," in *Deinstitutionalisation and People with Intellectual Disabilities: In and Out of Institutions,* eds. K. Johnson and R. Traustadottir (London: Jessica Kingsley, 2005).
19. Erving Goffman, *Asylums: Essays on the Social Situation of Mental Patients and Other Inmates* (Harmondsworth: Penguin, 1961).
20. K. Castles, "Nice Average Americans: Post-war Parents' Groups and the Defense of the Normal Family," in *Mental Retardation in America,* eds. S. Noll and J. Trent (New York: New York University Press, 2004).
21. Deborah C. Park and John P. Radford, "From the Case Files: Reconstructing a History of Involuntary Sterilization," *Disability and Society* 13, no. 3 (1998): 317–342.
22. K. Engwall, "Implications of Being Diagnosed as a 'Feeble-Minded' Woman," in *Gender and Disability Research in the Nordic Countries,* eds. Kristjana Kristiansen and Rannveig Traustadottir (Sweden: Studentlitteratur, 2004); Robert Edgerton, *The Cloak of Competence* (Berkeley: University of California Press, 1967); Tilley, Walmsley, Earle, and Atkinson, "The Silence Is Roaring."
23. Guðrún V. Stefánsdóttir and Eygló Ebba Hreinsdóttir, *It Shouldn't Be a Secret: Sterilisation of Women with Intellectual Disability in Iceland,* Nordic Network for Disability Research Conference, Reykjavik, Iceland, 27 May 2011.
24. Edgerton, *The Cloak of Competence,* 154.
25. Ibid., 155.
26. Ibid.
27. Tilley, Walmsley, Earle, and Atkinson, "The Silence Is Roaring."
28. Jones, *Social Hygiene.*
29. Tilley, Walmsley, Earle, and Atkinson, "The Silence Is Roaring"; A. Stansfield, I. Clare, and A. Holland, "The Sterilization of People with Intellectual Disabilities in England and Wales in the Period 1988–1999," *Journal of Intellectual Disability Research* 51, no. 8 (2007): 569–579.
30. Stansfield et al., "The Sterilization of People," 35.
31. Ibid., 36.
32. Tilley, Walmsley, Earle, and Atkinson, "The Silence Is Roaring."
33. Molly Ladd Taylor, "The 'Sociological Advantages' of Sterilization: Fiscal Policies and Feeble-Minded Women in Interwar Minnesota," in *Mental Retardation in America,* eds. Steven Noll and James Trent (New York: New York University Press, 2004), 281–302.
34. Stansfield et al., "The Sterilization of People."
35. L. Servais, R. Leach, D. Jacques, and J. P. Roussaux, "Sterilisation of Intellectually Disabled Women," *European Psychiatry* 19, no. 7 (2004): 428–432.

36. H. M. J. van Schrojenstein Lantman-de Valk, F. Rook, and M. A. Maaskant, "The Use of Contraception by Women with Intellectual Disabilities," *Journal of Intellectual Disability Research*, 55, no. 4 (April 2011): 434–440.
37. C. Hamilton, *New Zealand Law on the Sterilisation of Intellectually Disabled Women and Girls* (Unpublished report, 2011).
38. Hanna Björg Sigurjónsdóttir and Rannveig Traustadóttir, "Family Within a Family," in *Parents with Intellectual Disabilities,* eds. G. Llewellyn, R. Traustadottir, D. McConnell, and H. B. Sigurjonsdottir (West Sussex: Wiley Blackwell, 2010), 49–62, 50.
39. Michelle McCarthy, "Contraception and Women with Intellectual Disabilities," *Journal of Applied Research in Intellectual Disabilities*, 22, no. 4 (June 2009): 363–369; Michelle McCarthy, "'I Have the Jab So I Can't Be Blamed for Getting Pregnant': Contraception and Women with Learning Disabilities," *Women's Studies International Forum*, 32 (2009): 198–208; Michelle McCarthy, "Exercising Choice and Control—Women with Learning Disabilities and Contraception," *British Journal of Learning Disabilities*, 38 (November 2010): 293–302.
40. Tilley, Walmsley, Earle, and Atkison, "The Silence Is Roaring."
41. McCarthy, "Contraception and Women"; McCarthy, "I Have the Jab"; Susan Ledger, Jan Walmsley, Sarah Earle, and Elizabeth Tilley, "Contraceptive Decision-Making and Women with Learning Disabilities," *Sexualities* 19, nos. 5–6 (June 2016): 698–724.
42. Ledger, Walmsley, Earle, and Tilley, "Contraceptive Decision-Making."
43. Department of Health, *Valuing People Now: A New Three-Year Strategy for People with Learning Disabilities* (London: The Stationery Office, 2009), 2.
44. Erving Goffman, *Stigma: Notes on the Management of Spoiled Identity* (Harmondsworth: Penguin, 1963).
45. N. E. Bank-Mikkelson, "Modern Service Models," in *Changing Patterns in Residential Services for the Mentally Retarded* (Washington, DC: President's Committee on Mental Retardation, 1969).
46. Wolf Wolfensberger, *The Principle of Normalisation in Human Services* (Toronto: National Institute on Mental Retardation, 1972).
47. T. Buchner, O. Koenig, and G. Kremsner, "Intellectual Disabilities in Austria in the Twentieth and Twenty-First Centuries: Tracing the Historical and Ideological Roots and Dismantling the Current Locked State of Services for People with Intellectual Disabilities in Austria," in *Intellectual Disability in the Twentieth Century: Transnational Perspectives on People, Policy, and Practice,* eds. Jan Walmsley and Simon Jarrett (Bristol: Policy Press, forthcoming).

48. Daniel J. Kevles, *In the Name of Eugenics* (Boston, MA: Harvard University Press, 2004).
49. David G. Race, ed. *Leadership and Change in Human Services: Selected Readings from Wolf Wolfensberger* (London: Routledge, 2003).
50. Wolf Wolfensberger, "Extermination: Disabled People in Nazi Germany," *Disabled USA* 4, no. 2 (1980): 22–24, reprinted in Race, *Leadership and Change,* 190.
51. Race, *Leadership and Change,* 191–193.
52. Ibid., 186–187.
53. Mencap, *Death by Indifference* (London: Mencap, 2007). See also, Mencap, *Death by Indifference 74 Deaths and Counting: A Progress Report 5 Years On* (London: Mencap, 2012); Pauline Heslop, Peter Blair, Peter Fleming et al., *Confidential Inquiry into Premature Deaths of People with Intellectual Disabilities in the UK: A Population-Based Study* (Bristol: Norah Fry Research Centre, 2013).
54. Mazars, *Independent Review of Deaths of People with a Learning Disability or Mental Health Problem in Contact with Southern Health NHS Foundation Trust April 2011–March 2015* (2015). www.england.nhs.uk/south/wp-content/uploads/sites/6/2015/12/mazars-rep.pdf. Accessed 15 August 2017.
55. Wolf Wolfensberger, "A Call to Wake Up to the Beginning of a New Wave of 'Euthanasia' of Severely Impaired People," *Education and Training of the Mentally Retarded,* 15 (1980): 171–173, reprinted in Race, *Leadership and Change,* 189–191.
56. *A World Without Down's Syndrome?* (2016). BBC Two Television, 5 October. www.bbc.co.uk/programmes/b07ycbj5. Accessed 7 May 2017.
57. Philip Reilly, *Genetics, Law and Social Policy* (Boston: Harvard University Press, 1977).
58. Deborah R. Barnbaum, *The Ethics of Autism: Among Them But Not of Them* (Bloomington: Indiana University Press, 2008).
59. United Nations Convention on the Rights of Persons with Disabilities, *Inquiry Concerning the United Kingdom of Great Britain and Northern Ireland Carried Out by the Committee Under Article 6 of the Optional Protocol to the Convention: Report of the Committee* (Geneva: United Nations, 2016). www.ohchr.org/EN/HRBodies/CRPD/Pages/InquiryProcedure.aspx. Accessed 21 February 2017.
60. Kelley Johnson, Jan Walmsley with Marie Wolfe, *People with Intellectual Disabilities: Towards a Good Life?* (Bristol: The Policy Press, 2010).
61. John Rawls, *A Theory of Justice* (Oxford: Oxford University Press, 1999).
62. Peter Singer, *How Are We to Live? Ethics in an Age of Self-Interest* (Melbourne: Random House, 1993).

63. Goodey, *Learning Disability.*
64. Ibid., 13.
65. Ibid.
66. Ibid., 18.

CHAPTER 6

Sheltered Employment and Mental Health in Britain: Remploy c.1945–1981

Andy Holroyde

Introduction

The history of mental health provision is now firmly established as a major area of research. The traditional focus on the asylum has also now been complemented with examinations of what went on outside its walls, and the focus on the history of the institution, likewise, has been complemented by attempts to give voice to its service users.[1] Though research has tended to remain focused on the Victorian heyday of the asylum, studies which examine developments in mental health provision over the twentieth century have also appeared.[2] The process of deinstitutionalisation which occurred after the Second World War has attracted attention from both historians and social policy analysts.[3] Such considerations have focused on the key legislation passed in the period, particularly the Mental Health Act, 1959, and have presented an overall narrative of the move from residential institutions to community care, with a general conclusion that factors such as financial stringencies prevented the fulfilment of the objectives espoused by policymakers in this

A. Holroyde (✉)
University of Huddersfield, Huddersfield, UK
e-mail: Andrew.Holroyde@hud.ac.uk

S. J. Taylor and A. Brumby (eds.), *Healthy Minds in the Twentieth Century*, Mental Health in Historical Perspective,
https://doi.org/10.1007/978-3-030-27275-3_6

process.[4] As John Welshman noted, however, the roles of the various institutions which together formed this community of care in the post-war period, such as hostels, special schools and occupation centres, have remained largely neglected by historians.[5] Welshman himself began to remedy this with a preliminary exploration of the hostel system in the post-war period.[6] In the conclusion to this piece, Welshman called for further work examining the system of community care.[7] Responding to this call, this chapter seeks to provide a similar preliminary exploration of a further component of community care in the form of sheltered employment, chiefly that provided by Remploy.

The importance of employment to mental well-being and in the rehabilitation process of mental hospital patients has been noted by historians and social policy analysts. Employment within such institutional care for those with mental health conditions or learning disabilities has also been examined as part of the treatment provided. Historians have recognised the potential for such employment to be a positive experience for patients, providing, for example, a potential means to progress through the rehabilitation process, gain increasing independence and offer a source of friendship and informal care.[8] That employment could have a 'darker side as an instrument of punishment, imposed redemption and atonement, exploitation and a means of control' has also been recognised.[9] The provision of employment for patients once they had left such institutions was a key part of the transition to community living. Sheltered employment was an important aspect of this for those unable to secure work in open employment and represented something of a halfway house between the residential institution and the community in the promotion of 'healthy minds' for the mentally-ill.[10]

Remploy itself has received only scant attention from historians with limited references to its role in post-war disability employment provision. There were a range of voluntary organisations providing sheltered employment before the outbreak of the Second World War. Some schemes provided training or limited employment in residential settings such as St. Dunstan's, which was established in 1915 and did much to aid blind ex-servicemen, and the Star and Garter Home for Disabled Soldiers and Sailors, opened in 1916.[11] More ambitious schemes involved whole sheltered communities of disabled ex-servicemen, such as the Enham Village Centre settlement, which combined a rural environment with training and some employment.[12] The majority of schemes involved work in workshops or factories, the largest of which were the Lord Robert's Memorial Workshops. Established following the Boer War, they expanded during the First World War and at the end of 1919 employed over 600 men in several workshops around the country.[13] Though likely preferable to unemployment, such workshops could be less than ideal for workers and were run on very slight budgets owing to their reliance on continued public generosity.[14] Following the First World War, the British government did provide such charitable organisations with some limited financial support under the Ministry of Labour's 'Scheme of Grants'.[15] During the interwar period, the Ministry paid these grants to 'thirty separate enterprises', which Deborah Cohen suggested probably employed around 2000 workers, 'only a fraction of those who according to the government's figures needed work'.[16] At the close of the Second World War, there remained a number of voluntary providers of sheltered employment still in operation, though such provision was noted by the Ministry as being 'meagre and inadequate'.[17]

Remploy was established by the British government as part of the provision of the Disabled Persons (Employment) Act, 1944. The aim of the company was to provide sheltered employment on a national scale for those 'severely disabled people' who were considered unable to gain work in the open employment market. In a similar fashion to the nationalised industries, Remploy was run by a Board of Directors selected by the Ministry of Labour, who handled the day-to-day business of the company, while overall policy was directed by the Ministry. The company was intended to be as financially self-supporting as possible with any losses funded by the Treasury. A period of rapid expansion following the opening of the first Remploy factory in Bridgend in 1946 resulted in Remploy employing over 6000 disabled people across 91 factories by 1953.[18] The number of employees steadily grew over the subsequent decades with Remploy remaining the dominant provider of sheltered employment in the post-war period. This began to change in the 1980s, in response to the fundamental changes to the welfare state which occurred and the increasing desire to promote the inclusion of disabled people in open or 'mainstream' employment. Remploy factories began to be closed down and replaced by Remploy 'branches' on the high street which focused on providing employment services to support those with disabilities or health conditions into mainstream employment. Remploy's transition from sheltered employment to employment services provider was finally completed with the closure of the remaining Remploy factories in 2013. Further change occurred when, in April

2015, Remploy left government ownership. Continuing to provide specialist employment services, Remploy is, at the time of writing, owned by *Maximus*, an international provider of health and employment services, and Remploy employees themselves who hold a twenty per cent stake in the company.[19]

Though it was not the only form of sheltered employment available, with both voluntary organisations and Local Authorities also providing such services, Remploy was the majority provider. Owing to this and its place as the central government provider of sheltered employment, the company has, in contrast to the range of other organisations, left a significant imprint in the archives. This chapter will draw upon the wealth of material relating to the company located in the National Archives, as well as some archival material retained by the company itself. Remploy was initially called 'The Disabled Persons Employment Corporation', with its factories referred to as 'British Factories'. The name Remploy was in use from 1946 and officially adopted in 1949, though reference to the 'Corporation' continued for some years after this. In the interests of clarity, the term 'Remploy' will be used here. In terms of terminology in this chapter, the use of terms such as 'disability', 'disabled people', 'severely disabled people', 'Section I and II disabled people', 'mentally disabled people' and 'physically disabled people' solely reflects the specific historic bureaucratic categories applied to people during the period examined here and are not intended to reflect lived experience or personal/group identity. The term 'mentally disabled' is used frequently as a historic term which refers to a specific bureaucratic category which covered all forms of mental illness or learning disability and meant that a person was eligible for work in one of Remploy's factories. This chapter also includes occasional instances of use of what is now considered derogatory language in direct quotation from primary sources. This is done purely in the interests of historical accuracy in order to reflect the nomenclature of the period and is not intended to condone any current use of such terms.

This chapter will explore the role played by Remploy as the largest provider of sheltered employment in the provision of community care in the post-war period. The composition of Remploy's workforce has yet to be examined in detail and has thus largely been taken for granted by academics across disciplines as being simply 'disabled people' or 'severely disabled' people.[20] The popular viewpoint meanwhile, espoused by Remploy itself and regularly featured in media reports on the company, has suggested that Remploy was created to cater for those injured as a result of the Second World War.[21] There is a general assumption, therefore, that in the immediate post-war period Remploy catered solely for so-called physically disabled people. Yet by the mid-1980s, 40% of Remploy's employees were those with 'some form of mental or nervous handicap'.[22] This move from so-called physical to non-physical or 'mental' disability in the company's employees is understood by Remploy itself to be a key feature in the development of the company, yet there is no understanding of how this occurred beyond the assumption that the 1959 Mental Health Act instigated the change.[23] This development has similarly remained unexplored in considerations of Remploy and disability employment provision among academics. This chapter will therefore attempt to clarify the position of Remploy in the employment provision for mentally disabled people and to add this to our understanding of the development of sheltered employment in the post-war period. To do so it will consider first the impact of the 1959 Mental Health Act upon Remploy, to determine if this did indeed mark a turning point in the company as has been assumed. It will then consider the place of mentally disabled people within Remploy and whether the company adapted to reflect an increasing number of such employees.

The Impact of the 1959 Mental Health Act—A Turning Point?

The central legislative impetus for the move from institutional to community care for the mentally-ill was the Mental Health Act, 1959. One change instigated by the Act was that the former mental hospital patients became able to register as disabled in line with the Disabled Persons (Employment) Act and thereby become eligible for a place in a Remploy factory.[24] Though it has been suggested by historians that the legal changes imposed by the 1959 Act were not matched by practical application at the local level, the case of sheltered employment in this assessment has not been examined until now.[25] As noted, there has been an assumption that in the immediate post-war period, Remploy catered solely for the physically disabled until the 1959 Act resulted in the introduction of mentally disabled people. It is apparent, however, that Remploy had always included people designated as 'disabled' because of 'mental illness' or 'mental disability'. To understand this, it is first necessary to understand the process by which disabled people became eligible for a place in a Remploy factory.

Entry to Remploy involved a specific process which all potential workers had to follow. The first step to entering a Remploy factory was registering as a disabled person on the Disabled Persons' Employment Register.[26] This was the voluntary mechanism established by the Disabled Persons (Employment) Act, 1944, for gaining access to any of its provisions, including Remploy. The registration process involved a person fulfilling a number of criteria and certain exclusions applied. First, a person had to be considered disabled in accordance with the definition of the Act, which stated that:

> 'Disabled person'- means a person who, on account of injury, disease or congenital deformity, is substantially handicapped in obtaining or keeping employment, or in undertaking work on his own account, of a kind which apart from that injury, disease or deformity would be suited to his age, experience and qualifications.[27]

Beyond this general definition, the Act further stipulated that a person's disability must be likely to last for six months or more; that the person must be at least 14 years old; that they be resident in Great Britain; and that they be willing to undertake the training or employment offered.[28] Those disqualified from registration included prisoners, full-time hospital patients and those deemed to be of 'bad character'.[29] Mentally disabled people were therefore always included in the broad definition of disability contained in the Act. There were, however, some further exclusions which applied to disabled people who were subject to treatment under the Lunacy and Mental Treatments Acts.[30] The scope of such exclusions was given further consideration by the Ministry of Labour in 1945, following calls from the Board of Control and the London County Council for clarity regarding whether those 'mental defectives' receiving treatment, particularly in the case of those living outside institutions, were eligible for registration or not.[31] Following a process of consultation between the Board of Control, the Ministry of Health and the Ministry of Labour, it was finally agreed that registration was possible for those under treatment or supervision under the Mental Deficiency Act, provided such persons were considered likely to be able to gain and keep employment.[32] Exclusion from registration continued to apply to those who were resident in mental hospitals or institutions unless they were individually authorised to be absent on licence.[33]

Having registered upon the Disabled Persons' Employment Register, a disabled person was then assessed and designated as being either

'Section I' or 'Section II'. Section I disabled people were those considered able to secure work in open employment and represented the majority of those registered. The Section II designation applied to those considered too 'severely disabled' to access open employment, and thereby as requiring sheltered employment provision. Those designated as Section II were therefore eligible for a place in Remploy, and it was from this pool of disabled people that Remploy could recruit its factory workers. Eligibility was therefore determined on the basis of the impact of a person's disability upon their employment prospects, and as such, mentally disabled people were able to register and become eligible for Remploy. The inclusion of such cases in Remploy was always expected, as the Ministry of Labour made clear when considering the issue of placing those with 'psychiatric disorders' in employment in 1945.[34]

At no time in its existence did Remploy employ all Section II, and therefore theoretically eligible, disabled people, but rather selected a limited number of employees from this pool of potential recruits. As Remploy began to expand in the late 1940s, it is apparent that Remploy did indeed include those with mental disabilities within its disabled workforce. Unfortunately, there is no breakdown of what was termed the 'disability mix' within the company extant for the early period of Remploy's operation. Some localised examples do attest to the inclusion of mentally disabled people in the workforce, with the Halifax Remploy factory including an individual with 'low mentality' among its employees in 1948, and with the Barking Remploy factory noting that it had a dozen employees suffering 'Neurosis' among its workers.[35] Furthermore, a guide for Remploy factory managers published and distributed by the company in 1949 made reference to those with 'mental disabilities' as one category of disabled employee factory managers were dealing with.[36]

A full company breakdown of its disabled employees comes from December 1954, by which time Remploy had completed its initial factory expansion, with 91 factories in operation employing some 6433 disabled people.[37] Of these disabled employees, some 530 were classified as having a 'mental disability' in terms of neurosis, psychoneurosis or 'nervous or mental disorders'.[38] Remploy was therefore employing a significant number of people, a little over 8% of its workforce, with mental disabilities five years prior to the passing of the 1959 Act. It is apparent therefore that the 1959 Act did not introduce mentally disabled people into Remploy and that the assumption that the company catered exclusively for the physically disabled in the immediate post-war period does not reflect the reality.

The question then is what impact the 1959 Act did have upon Remploy. During discussion of the Act in the House of Commons, anxiety was expressed by the Labour MP Edward Mallalieu, when querying what was to become of those deinstitutionalised in terms of employment and whether there would be specialist sheltered employment for such cases 'on the Remploy model'.[39] In the House of Lords, the following year, it was suggested that Remploy should take a central role in providing sheltered employment for those deinstitutionalised.[40] Remploy was not something that required setting-up, it was already in the community and was already employing people considered 'severely disabled' due to mental illness or disability. One might be forgiven, therefore, for assuming that they would be greatly utilised as part of the move to community care following the 1959 Act. Remploy later described how it had taken a 'fair share of this burden' in terms of the policy of deinstitutionalisation, so that by 1964 '10% or our total disabled employees were suffering from mental disabilities'.[41] However, when compared with the 8% of such cases a decade earlier, it is apparent that the Act did not lead to an immediate sea change in terms of recruitment policy and a sudden influx of such cases within Remploy, with an increase of only 2% over 10 years. Indeed, by December 1959, the figure was already approaching 9%.[42]

With Remploy already including a significant proportion of workers with mental disabilities, it appears that the focus for the company following the passing of the Act was on a cautious consideration of how the company might cater for the newly eligible former mental hospital patients who may have had more 'severe' mental health conditions than the company had yet been asked to accommodate. As the Executive Director of Remploy noted, it had previously been the policy in Remploy that 'serious mental cases were not employed'.[43] The initial response to the 1959 Act was therefore the undertaking of an experiment in employing 'serious mental cases' in the form of mental hospital patients suffering from schizophrenia. The experiment was conducted in 1960 in conjunction with the Ministry of Labour and the Medical Research Council.[44] This involved the employment of a small number of such 'serious' cases across a group of factories.[45] Thus, by April 1960, there were three such persons employed in the Croydon Remploy factory and one in the Barking factory, with two more awaiting employment in the Park Royal factory and Southampton factory, respectively.[46]

The following month saw the extension of the experiment with a further small intake at the Bermondsey factory and the inclusion of two former patients from the Long Grove Hospital at the Radcliffe factory.[47] At the meeting of the Remploy Board of Directors in which the experiment was discussed, one member expressed her surprise 'that we were employing schizophrenic patients in our factories'.[48] It was explained by the Executive Director that this was part of a limited experiment and that the 'persons recruited by Remploy were very carefully selected'.[49] This selection appears to have included advice from medical experts, as well as a series of interviews and discussions with several management levels within Remploy, with careful consideration of each case.[50] The Managing Director noted that those employed were 'doing very well'.[51] Similarly, the Executive Director was able to claim that those recruited 'had proved to be very good workers'.[52] The representative of the Ministry of Labour at the meeting further explained that the Minister himself had received a special report on the progress of the experiment thus far and was 'very pleased and heartened with the action taken'.[53] Indeed, the experiment was referenced in the House of Commons in July 1961 with Mr William Morgan, the Conservative MP for Denbigh noting:

> Remploy factories do not remain static in their attitude to employment. I was gratified to learn from a recent report that the Remploy factories have, by arrangement with my right hon. Friend the Minister of Labour, taken in a small number of patients suffering from the effects of schizophrenia. This effort to give mentally disordered persons a place in the working life of the community deserves every sympathy and encouragement. The rehabilitation of these particularly unfortunate disabled persons is a challenging experiment, and it must be a satisfaction to us all that the results, according to the report, have so far been very encouraging.[54]

Such 'experimentation' in using employment to make 'sick' minds 'healthy' was not limited to Remploy, with sheltered employment run by Local Authorities and voluntary institutions also responding to the change in eligibility for registration brought on by the 1959 Act. In 1960, for example, the City of Leeds introduced a sheltered works programme in its parks department, while the following year the Industrial Therapy Organisation in Bristol launched an 'experimental scheme' providing 'special supervision' to a group of ex-mental hospital patients in open industry.[55] In addition to this, the Industrial Therapy Organisation established a car-wash scheme which 'was operated entirely by mental patients, many of whom had been in psychiatric hospitals for a number of years'.[56] In a report on the scheme by the National Advisory Council on the Employment of the Disabled (NACED), established by the Disabled Persons (Employment) Act to oversee the progress of its provision, the car wash was 'running at a profit and well patronised by the Bristol public' with the suggestion that this had contributed to a positive change 'in the attitudes of the public towards the mentally disordered'.[57] As with Remploy, it was noted that for all such schemes 'the workers involved were specially selected patients'.[58]

The Mental Health Act did not, therefore, lead to a sea change in who was recruited by Remploy and did not instigate a sudden influx of former mental hospital patients into the company. Its impact in the immediate term was rather a limited experiment with carefully selected cases of those newly eligible for Remploy. The Act does appear, however, to have supported an existing longer-term trend of increasing numbers of mentally disabled people registering upon the Disabled Persons Employment Register and thereby increasing the proportion of such cases within Remploy's recruitment pool. In 1963, people with 'mental illness or mental handicap' represented 14% of the Section II register; by 1973, this had increased to 20% and by 1978 had reached 25%.[59] This increase was similarly reflected in the proportion of those with mental disabilities employed by Remploy. By 1974, the proportion of employees with mental disabilities in Remploy had increased to 17%, making it the largest disability 'grouping' in the company, and by 1978 had increased again to 20%.[60] This trend was well recognised by both Remploy and the government. During a debate in the House of Commons on the employment of disabled people in 1972, it was noted that 'mental and nervous conditions are of growing significance'.[61] In its investigation of sheltered employment the following year, the Department of Employment, previously the Ministry of Labour, suggested this trend was a result of both 'modern techniques of care and attention' by which 'mentally handicapped or mentally ill people are enjoying a longer and full life' as well as 'present mental health policies…aimed at minimising in-patient treatment'.[62] The result was that 'more and more mentally handicapped and mentally ill people are becoming available for sheltered employment'.[63]

A significant change clearly occurred in Remploy's disability mix over the period considered in this chapter, with a steady increase in the number of mentally disabled people as a proportion of both those employed by Remploy and in terms of those eligible to apply for a place with the company.[64] The Mental Health Act, 1959, and the policy of deinstitutionalisation are therefore best understood as contributors to a longer-term trend in terms of eligibility for sheltered employment, which Remploy steadily increasingly drew upon.

Mental Disability Within Remploy

With Remploy employing an increasing number of mentally disabled people over the course of the period examined in this chapter, it is important to consider the impact such a change had upon the company. This chapter will now consider the place of those with mental disabilities in Remploy and whether the company adapted to reflect the changes in who it was employing.

As previously noted, Remploy did not simply employ all those eligible under the Disabled Persons (Employment) Act, designated as being Section II. Rather, the company selected those it wished from the available Section II pool of candidates. From the beginning, the Remploy Board of Directors were clear that they felt that the primary purpose of Remploy was to provide 'genuine employment' and establish a viable long-term business for its severely disabled employees. There was to be no place for either charity or simple occupational therapy.[65] The 'treatment' or 'rehabilitation' provided by Remploy was in terms of the understood benefits of worthwhile employment for the individual. The aim of the company was 'to provide productive and worthwhile work' in an environment which resembled a 'normal' industrial operation as closely as possible.[66] The 1956 report of the *Committee of Inquiry on the Rehabilitation, Training and Resettlement of Disabled Persons* (Piercy Report), established to review the progress of the provisions of the Disabled Persons (Employment) Act, emphasised the importance of productivity and the concept of genuine employment in distinguishing sheltered employment provision from purely occupational welfare.[67] The report of the *Royal Commission on the Law Relating to Mental Illness and Mental Deficiency* (Percy Commission) the following year endorsed the application of this principle 'with regard to mentally handicapped or disabled patients'.[68] Sheltered employment provision such as Remploy was therefore to provide employment for those capable of undertaking work with a degree of productivity. The chief aspect considered in recruitment to Remploy was not therefore a person's disability per se, but rather the potential productivity of the applicant. In short, Remploy factory managers were primarily concerned with recruiting the most productive workers from the available Section II pool of candidates, regardless of the person's particular disability. As such, those with mental disabilities were considered for work in a Remploy factory by this same measure, with only those capable of undertaking the factory work required being recruited and retained by the company.

In following this principle, Remploy employed workers with a wide range of disabilities. The records for the company reveal that consideration was regularly given to potential issues involved in the employment of people with different disabilities. In terms of mentally disabled people specifically, there were regular questions raised about the benefits of integration. The notion that mentally disabled people should be segregated within sheltered employment had been raised from the very beginning of Remploy, with consideration about the placing of 'psycho-neurotics' in 1945.[69] There was broad agreement within the Ministry of Labour at that time that in such cases 'segregation is undesirable'.[70] Such a policy was subsequently adopted by Remploy, with the only case of segregation along the lines of disability being the establishment of a number of dedicated Tuberculosis (TB) factories owing to the danger of infection. As such, in the case of Remploy, mentally disabled people both before and after the passing of the 1959 Mental Health Act were not segregated.

In the wider field of sheltered employment, things were not as clear-cut. Unlike Remploy, sheltered employment provided by voluntary organisations could often be limited to particular groups of disabled people. This reflected the various purposes and 'causes' to which these organisations were devoted. In the most obvious example, sheltered employment in TB sanatoria was, of course, available only for those with TB. Similarly, those sheltered workshops run by the British Legion provided only for the ex-servicemen which the charity was established to support, while the workshop run by the Ayrshire Society for the Deaf, as its name suggests, provided sheltered employment only for the deaf.[71] In the case of mental illness, in 1945 only one organisation explicitly focused on this group, Thermega Limited, which provided employment for 36 disabled men suffering from 'Neurosis, psychosis and associated diseases'.[72] By 1965, a Ministry of Labour list of 'approved independent charitable sheltered employment providers' included several which were explicitly devoted to mentally disabled people. This included the Industrial Therapy Organisation which employed 68 'mainly mentally handicapped men and women' and the Camphill Village Trust, which employed 183 'mentally handicapped men and women' across three sites.[73] In terms of Local Authorities too, the NACED noted in 1965 that several Authorities had followed Leeds in providing sheltered employment programmes specifically aimed at mentally disabled people.[74]

The policy view remained, however, that integration was generally preferable wherever possible. This view was endorsed by the Secretary of State for Employment and Productivity in 1968, when he expressed his belief that 'sheltered workshops should cater as Remploy does, for both the mentally and physically handicapped'.[75] This was reiterated under the following government in 1971, with the Under-Secretary of State for Employment replying to a query regarding the possibility of providing sheltered employment exclusively for the 'mentally handicapped', that 'sheltered work is generally best provided in workshops catering for all kinds of severely disabled people'.[76] The Department of Employment's detailed examination of the sheltered employment field in 1973 argued too that it was desirable that such provision avoided 'arrangements whereby people are segregated into particular categories of disability' and made 'integrated arrangements as far as it is possible to do so'.[77] The Department recognised, however, 'that broad policy contains certain areas of difficulty and uncertainty, especially in the fields of mental handicap and mental illness; and there may sometimes be good reason for separate measures for particular disabilities in certain circumstances'.[78] Such a case occurred in 1976, with a proposal, at the request from the Department of Employment, for Remploy to open a factory entirely for some 90 mentally-ill patients in Surrey.[79] This was not, however, due to any belief that this was inherently preferable; rather, it was owing to practicalities and location.[80] The issue being that there were 100 such cases in hospitals in the Epsom area all deemed to be 'suitable for sheltered employment'.[81] Rather than 'dispersing them around the country, with all the problems that would be involved in finding work and accommodation', the better option was believed to be to 'open a factory, solely for them in the immediate location'.[82] This project was not to come to fruition and it remained the case that mentally disabled people remained integrated into Remploy as policy. Arguably, this policy of integration may have had a positive effect on the minds of those suffering from mental illnesses, by offering them regular employment and the opportunity to assimilate into a broader community.

One consequence of this policy of integration was that mentally disabled people would have to essentially 'fit-in' with the normal 'flow' of a Remploy factory in the same way as any other disabled employee. The question is therefore whether the increasing proportion of employees with mental disabilities resulted in any changes to the way Remploy operated. In 1964, Remploy's personnel director spoke at an international conference on social psychiatry in London on the topic of 'practical problems on the employment of the mentally handicapped'.[83] Such discussions were not unique to considerations of mental disability, with regular reflections from the company on employment 'issues' relating to a range of disabilities within the company occurring throughout the period. However, the increasing number of mentally disabled employees within Remploy does seem to have led to greater consideration of the implications raised, with a belief that this offered particular challenges for factory management.

In 1974, responding to concerns expressed by a group of factory managers, it was decided by Remploy to undertake 'teach-ins' across the company, with factory managers and doctors invited for group discussion and instruction in order 'to increase our skill in handling mentally disabled people'.[84] At a meeting of the Remploy Board of Directors discussing the 'teach-ins', the Managing Director 'stressed the importance of these, with the increasing numbers of mentally disabled in Remploy, and the need for even experienced factory managers to have more guidance'.[85] It was explained that the key point raised during the teach-ins 'which has already come across very forcibly (and which has been raised before many times by works managers) is the need to improve the ratio of supervisory staff to disabled employees, especially where mentally disabled people are concerned'.[86] This question of additional supervision appears to have been the main conclusion from the sessions, with no commitment to take further action.[87] The only hint of any notion of instigating systemic change in the way Remploy operated was a remark by one Board member that having attended one of these teach-ins, 'he had become very much aware that the Company might have to change some points of its basic policy of employment if mental illness were to be catered for'.[88]

There was, therefore, to be no meaningful consideration of fundamental change to Remploy until the early 1980s with two internal reports examining the issue. The first of these was a wide-ranging report considering the fundamental purpose of Remploy and its 'criteria of success'.[89] As part of its findings, the report noted that since its establishment, the key development in terms of Remploy's recruitment pool was the significant change 'from physical to mental disability'.[90] It then echoed the conclusions from the 'teach-ins', claiming that there remained a 'generally held view' in the company that an 'increase in the numbers of supervisory staff to disabled employees' was necessary in order 'to maintain an acceptable level of productivity and efficiency'.[91] The recommendation of the report was that 'a limit should be placed on the numbers of mentally disabled; if this cannot be controlled serious consideration would have to be given to establishing separate units within Remploy for the employment of the mentally disabled'.[92] As a result of this report, a working party was formed to fully examine the issue of the so-called disability mix in Remploy. The report explained:

> The chief aspect of disability mix on which Remploy Managers have fairly firm opinions is that of mental disability. Maintaining an acceptable balance between employees with mental and nervous disabilities and those with physical handicaps is regarded as a major problem and managers are keenly interested therefore in trends in disability mix.[93]

The report noted the expectation that the trend of an increase in the 'proportion of mentally disabled' would continue.[94] Ultimately, however, it rejected the idea of establishing any limit or set quota, highlighting that there was already a 'smaller proportion of mentally handicapped people' working in Remploy than were on the Disabled Persons Register.[95] The report further argued that while there were concerns expressed by some factory managers, there were many examples where there were no issues with integration within factories.[96] The report concluded that it was ultimately up to factory managers to deal with any issues which arose on a case-by-case basis. The solutions proposed were focused on supporting this with better training for managers.[97] This was not to be the end of the issue, with the report suggesting further consideration would be needed regarding how the company should readjust to reflect the increasing proportion of mentally disabled employees.[98] Such considerations were to wait until later in the decade when changes in the welfare state, manufacturing industry and perceptions of sheltered employment itself were to lead to more fundamental changes to Remploy. While concerns were frequently expressed, therefore, and the issue of changes to Remploy examined carefully, action in the period considered in this chapter was limited to the offer of more support for factory management to manage their employees effectively.

Conclusions

Contrary to both the popular and scholarly understanding of Remploy, this chapter has illustrated that the inclusion of mentally disabled people within the company's disabled workforce was not a sudden result of the 1959 Mental Health Act but was a feature of the company from its very beginning. It was always expected that Remploy would employ those considered 'severely disabled' in line with the Disabled Persons (Employment) Act, 1944 owing to mental illness or disability and it is apparent that they did so. The promotion of 'healthy minds' through productive work in Remploy was thus available to mentally disabled people. The immediate impact of the 1959 Act was the limited inclusion of some of the more 'serious' cases of mental hospital patients the company might be expected to employ, with similar experiments undertaken by other organisations. The most significant effect of the Act was in supporting an existing trend in increasing numbers of mentally disabled people entering Remploy's recruitment pool. While this change in the company's 'disability mix' did provoke some concern among factory management, there was to be no serious consideration of whether it justified a fundamental rethink of how Remploy operated until the early 1980s. As such, mentally disabled people in Remploy were recruited and employed in the factories on the same basis as all disabled workers. Individual productivity and how well a person could 'fit-in' with the operations of the given factory would determine their access to Remploy. In offering such conclusions, the nature of this chapter as a preliminary examination bears repeating. Further research into the place of sheltered employment within the process of deinstitutionalisation and into the experiences of mentally disabled people across the range of sheltered employment providers would contribute enormously to our understanding of how employment was considered to aid in the promotion of 'healthy minds'.

Notes

1. Peter Bartlett and David Wright, eds., *Outside the Walls of the Asylum: The History of Care in the Community 1750–2000* (London: Athlone Press, 1999); Lindsay Brigham et al., eds., *Crossing Boundaries: Change and*

Continuity in the History of Learning Disability (Kidderminster: BILD Publications, 2000).

2. Mathew Thomson, *The Problem of Mental Deficiency: Eugenics, Democracy, and Social Policy in Britain, c. 1870–1959* (Oxford: Clarendon Press, 1998); Pamela Dale and Joseph Melling, eds., *Mental Illness and Learning Disability Since 1850* (Abingdon: Routledge, 2006).
3. Kathleen Jones, *Mental Health and Social Policy 1845–1959* (London: Routledge & Kegan Paul, 1960); Kathleen Jones, *A History of the Mental Health Services* (London: Routledge & Kegan Paul, 1972); Julian Leff, ed., *Care in the Community: Illusion or Reality?* (Chichester: Wiley, 1997); Helen Lester and Jon Glasby, *Mental Health Policy and Practice* (2nd edition) (Basingstoke: Palgrave Macmillan, 2010); Kelley Johnson and Rannveig Traustadottir, eds., *Deinstitutionalization and People with Intellectual Disabilities: In and Out of Institutions* (London: Jessica Kingsley, 2005).
4. Lester and Glasby, *Mental Health Policy and Practice*, 30–31; John Welshman, "Rhetoric and Reality: Community Care in England and Wales 1948–74," in *Outside the Walls of the Asylum*, eds. Bartlett and Wright; John Carrier and Ian Kendall, "Evolution of Policy," in *Care in the Community*, ed. Leff, 3–20; Jones, *Mental Health and Social Policy*, 153–206; Jones, *A History of the Mental Health Services*, 306–352; Alan Roulstone and Simon Prideaux, *Understanding Disability Policy* (Bristol: Policy Press, 2012), 36–39.
5. John Welshman, "Inside the Walls of the Hostel, 1940–74," in *Mental Illness and Learning Disability Since 1850*, eds. Dale and Melling, 200.
6. Ibid., 200–223.
7. Ibid., 219–220.
8. Ibid., 216–217.
9. Ibid.
10. The National Archives (Henceforth TNA), LAB 20/1429, Department of Employment, *Sheltered Employment: A Draft Consultative Document* (October 1973), 11–14.
11. For more on these, see Julie Anderson, *War, Disability and Rehabilitation in Britain: 'Soul of a Nation'* (Manchester: Manchester University Press, 2011), 49–55; Julie Anderson and Neil Pemberton, "Walking Alone: Aiding the War and Civilian Blind in the Inter-War Period," *European Review of History* 14, no. 4 (2007): 459–479.
12. For these schemes, see *Village Settlements for Disabled Ex-Service Men Scheme*, October 1917; "Village Settlements for the Disabled," *The Lancet*, 3 November 1917; "Reconstruction: Village Settlements for Disabled Ex-Service Men," *Westminster Gazette*, 9 November 1917—all in the National Archives TNA, PIN 15/34; Village Centres Council,

First Annual Report 1919, TNA, PIN 15/37; *Minutes of Third Meeting, Committee on Employment of Severely Disabled Ex-Service Men* (20 October 1920), TNA, PIN 15/36.

13. TNA, LAB 20/56 R.D.9, *Inter-Departmental Committee on the Rehabilitation and Resettlement of Disabled Persons: Note by the Ministry of Pensions*.
14. See Deborah Cohen, *The War Come Home: Disabled Veterans in Britain and Germany 1914–1939* (Los Angeles: University of California Press, 2001), 112–114, for criticisms of sheltered employment generally. Anderson, *Soul of a Nation*, 27–28 presents a more positive assessment.
15. TNA, CAB 24/123/79, *Cabinet Summary of the Report of the Committee Appointed to Consider the Employment of Severely Disabled Ex-Service Men (with special reference to Lords Roberts Memorial Workshops)* (25 May 1921); TNA, PIN 15/34, *Memo by Finance Department as to the Financial Position of the Lord Roberts Memorial Workshops*; Cohen, *The War Come Home*, 44–46; Sir Smedley Crooke to Mr. E. Brown, *Hansard* (22 December 1938), vol. 342 cc. 3101-3w.
16. Cohen, *The War Come Home*, 45–46.
17. TNA, LAB 20/173, NACED: Sheltered Employment Committee, *Report to the National Advisory Council on the Employment of the Disabled*, N.A.C. 9 (10 May 1945).
18. TNA, BM 10/1, *The Disabled Persons Employment Corporation Limited Later Remploy Limited: A Review of the Working of the Company During Its First Seven Years* (March 1953), 34.
19. Remploy, "Our Business." https://www.remploy.co.uk/about-us/our-business.
20. Jameel Hampton, "Discovering Disability: The General Classes of Disabled People and the Classic Welfare State, 1948–1964," *The Historian* 75, no. 1 (March 2013): 80; Linda Bryder, *Below the Magic Mountain: A Social History of Tuberculosis in Twentieth-Century Britain* (Oxford: Oxford University Press, 1988), 237; Sue Wheatcroft, *Worth Saving: Disabled Children During the Second World War* (Manchester: Manchester University Press, 2013), 168; Mark Hyde, "Sheltered and Supported Employment in the 1990s: The Experiences of Disabled Workers in the UK," *Disability & Society* 13, no. 2 (July 1998): 200; Paul Bridgen and R. Lowe, *Welfare Policy Under the Conservatives 1951–1964* (London: Public Record Office Handbooks, 1998), 262–263; Helen Bolderson, *Social Security, Disability and Rehabilitation: Conflicts in the Development of Social Policy 1914–1946* (London: Jessica Kingsley, 1991), 109; Eda Topliss, *Provision for the Disabled* (Oxford: Wiley-Blackwell, 1979), 56; Matthias Reiss, *Blind Workers Against Charity: The National League of the Blind of Great Britain and Ireland, 1893–1970* (London: Palgrave

Macmillan, 2015), 139; Julie Anderson, "'Turned into Taxpayers': Paraplegia, Rehabilitation and Sport at Stoke Mandeville, 1944–56," *Journal of Contemporary History* 38, no. 3 (July 2003): 469; Colin Barnes, *Disabled People in Britain and Discrimination* (London: C. Hurst & Company, 2000), 71; Anne Borsay, *Disability and Social Policy in Britain Since 1750* (Basingstoke: Palgrave, 2005), 135; Pat Thane, *Foundations of the Welfare State* (2nd edition) (London: Routledge, 1996), 225.

21. Remploy "Who We Are," Remploy Website 2017. http://www.remploy.co.uk/info/20124/find_out_more/72/who_we_are; Remploy "Remploy's Journey," Remploy Website 2017. http://www.remploy.co.uk/downloads/file/141/remploys_journeypdf; Nikki Fox, "What Are Remploy Workers Doing Now?" *BBC News* (31 November 2014). http://www.bbc.co.uk/news/uk-29843567; Jason Beattie, "Hundreds of Axes Disabled Workers Still Jobless Two Years After Remploy Factory Closures," *Mirror*, 5 January 2015. http://www.mirror.co.uk/news/uk-news/hundreds-axed-disabled-workers-still-4919835; ITV Report, "Remploy's History as Specialist Disabled Employer Remembered as Final Factories Close," 31 October 2013. http://www.itv.com/news/2013-10-31/final-remploy-factory-closes/; Historic England, "Disability History: Disability, Rehabilitation and Work" (2017). https://historicengland.org.uk/research/inclusive-heritage/disability-history/1945-to-the-present-day/disability-rehabilitation-and-work/.
22. TNA, BM 10/53, Remploy Limited, *Remploy Facts* (September 1986); TNA, BM 10/55, Remploy Limited, *Who We Are* (1994); TNA, BM 10/52, Remploy Limited, *Remploy: Company Profile* (1997); TNA, BM 10/57, Remploy Limited, *Remploy: Planning Our Future* (1998).
23. TNA, BM 10/2, R. E. Benjamin, *A Brief Outline of the Birth and Early Development of Remploy Limited* (May 1979), 26.
24. The Act had received an amendment in 1958, TNA, BM 10/2, Benjamin, *Brief Outline of the Birth and Early Development of Remploy*, 26.
25. Welshman, "Inside the Walls of the Hostel," 210.
26. Borsay, *Disability and Social Policy*, 135; Topliss, *Provision for the Disabled*, 49.
27. *Disabled Persons (Employment) Act (1944)* para 1.
28. *Disabled Persons (Employment) Act (1944)* para 7; Bolderson, *Social Security*, 117.
29. Bolderson, *Social Security*, 117. See also TNA, LAB 20/109.
30. Ibid.
31. TNA, LAB 20/212, Board of Control, *Letter to Miss Hill MOL* (27.11.1945); TNA, LAB 20/212, MOL, *Letter to Mr. Bleakley, Board of Control* (8 December 1945).
32. TNA, LAB 20/212, MOL, *Disabled Persons (Employment)Act, 1944: Register of Disabled Persons* (11 December 1945).

33. TNA, LAB 20/212, MOL, *Disabled Persons (Employment) Act, 1944: Registration of Patients of Mental Hospitals* (13 December 1950); TNA, BM 3/7, Remploy Limited, *Letter from Personnel Manager to St. Lawrence's Hospital Management Committee* (6 January1958).
34. TNA, LAB 20/173, NACED Sheltered Employment Committee, *Employment of Persons Suffering from Psychiatric Disorders* (S.E.C. 9).
35. TNA, LAB 20/444, The Disabled Persons Employment Corporation Limited, *Executive Director Report 36: Appendix B* (18 November 1948); *Fourth Report from the Select Committee on Estimates* (April 1952) (162), Annex 9, 100.
36. TNA, BM 5/9, Remploy Limited, *Factory Manager's Guide* (1949).
37. TNA, BM 8/23, Remploy Limited, *Managing Director's Report No. 30* (16 March 1955), *Appendix L, The Disabled Persons Employment Corporation Limited later Remploy Limited: A Review of the Working of the Company during its First Seven Years* (March 1953), 34.
38. TNA, BM 8/23, Remploy Limited, *Managing Director's Report No. 30* (16 March 1955), *Appendix L.*
39. Mr. Mallalieu (26 January 1959), *Hansard*, vol. 598, cc. 822.
40. Lord Stonham (28 November 1960), *Hansard*, vol. 226 cc. 919-20.
41. TNA, BM 10/48, Remploy Limited, *Company Objectives and Criteria of Financial Success* (7 January 1980), *Appendix No. 7*; TNA, BM 10/2, Benjamin, *A Brief Outline of the Birth and Early Development of Remploy Limited*, 26.
42. TNA, BM 8/32, Remploy Limited, *Managing Director Report No. 85: Appendix K* (9 March 1960).
43. TNA, BM 8/2, Remploy Limited, *Minutes of the One Hundred and Thirty-First Meeting of the Board of Directors* (15 May 1957).
44. TNA, BM 10/2, Benjamin, *A Brief Outline*, 26; TNA, BM 8/32, Remploy Limited, *Report of the Managing Director, No. 88* (May 1960).
45. TNA, BM 10/2, Benjamin, *A Brief Outline*, 26.
46. TNA, BM 8/32, Remploy Limited, *Report of the Managing Director, No. 86* (April 1960).
47. TNA, BM 8/32, Remploy Limited, *Supplement to Managing Director's Report No. 87* (11 May 1960); TNA, BM 8/32, Remploy Limited, *Report of the Managing Director, No. 88* (May 1960).
48. TNA, BM 8/2, Remploy Limited, *Minutes of the One Hundred and Sixty-Fifth Meeting of the Board of Directors* (18 May 1960).
49. Ibid.
50. TNA, BM 8/32, Remploy Limited, *Report of the Managing Director, No. 88* (May 1960).
51. TNA, BM 8/32, Remploy Limited, *Report of the Managing Director, No. 86* (April 1960).

52. TNA, BM 8/2, Remploy Limited, *Minutes of the One Hundred and Sixty-Fifth Meeting of the Board of Directors* (18 May 1960).
53. TNA, BM 8/2, Remploy Limited, *Minutes of the One Hundred and Sixty-Fifth Meeting of the Board of Directors* (18 May 1960).
54. Mr W.G. Morgan, *Hansard* (12 July 1961), vol. 644 cc. 486.
55. TNA, LAB 20/1429, DE, *Sheltered Employment: A Draft Consultative Document* (October 1973), 13–14; TNA, LAB 20/1211, NACED Sheltered Employment Committee: *Provision of Sheltered Employment for the Mentally Ill in Private Firms: S.E.C. 114* (November 1965).
56. TNA, LAB 20/1211, NACED, *Minutes of Meeting* (19 January 1966).
57. Ibid.
58. Ibid.
59. TNA, BM 10/48, Remploy Limited, *Company Objectives and Criteria of Financial Success* (7 January 1980), *Appendix No. 7.*
60. Ibid.
61. Mr. Dudley Smith (21 June 1972), *Hansard*, vol. 839 c. 680.
62. TNA, LAB 20/1429, DE, *Sheltered Employment: A Draft Consultative Document* (October 1973), 33–34.
63. Ibid., 33–34.
64. TNA, BM 10/48, Remploy Limited, *Company Objectives and Criteria of Financial Success* (7 January 1980), 21.
65. TNA, BM 10/1, *The Disabled Persons Employment Corporation Limited Later Remploy Limited: A Review of the Working of the Company During Its First Seven Years* (March 1953), 47.
66. Ibid.
67. *Report of the Committee of Inquiry on The Rehabilitation Training and Resettlement of Disabled Persons* (Cmd. 9883) (November 1956), House of Commons Parliamentary Papers Online; Topliss, *Provision for the Disabled*, 55–57; Reiss, *Blind Workers Against Charity*, 138–140.
68. *Report of the Royal Commission on the Law Relating to Mental Illness and Mental Deficiency* (Cmd. 169) (May 1957), House of Commons Parliamentary Papers Online, 225–226.
69. TNA, LAB 20/173, NACED Sheltered Employment Committee, *Employment of Persons Suffering from Psychiatric Disorders (S.E.C. 9).*
70. Ibid.
71. TNA, LAB 20/173, Committee on Sheltered Employment, *Undertakings Providing Employment for the Severely Disabled Other Than Those at Present Included in the Ministry of Labour and National Service Scheme of Grants S.E.C. 2* (1945).
72. Ibid.
73. TNA, LAB 20/1073, NACED Sheltered Employment Committee, *Approved Arrangements Made by Local Authorities for Providing Sheltered*

Employment for Severely Disabled Sighted Persons (1965); TNA, LAB 20/1429, Department of Employment, *Sheltered Employment: A Draft Consultative Document* (October 1973), 21.

74. TNA, LAB 20/1073, NACED Sheltered Employment Committee, *Provision of Sheltered Employment by Local Authorities and Voluntary Bodies: S.E.C. 111* (November 1965).
75. Mr. Fernyhough (9 July 1968), *Hansard*, vol. 768 c. 48w.
76. Mr. Dudley Smith (30 July 1971), *Hansard,* vol. 822 cc. 180-1w
77. TNA, LAB 20/1429, DE, *Sheltered Employment: A Draft Consultative Document* (October 1973), 47.
78. Ibid.
79. TNA, BM 8/79, Remploy Limited, *Minutes of the Three Hundred and Thirty-Eighth Meeting of the Board of Directors* (19 February 1976).
80. Ibid.
81. Ibid.
82. Ibid.
83. TNA, BM 6/10, *Remploy News, No. 63* (Autumn 1964).
84. TNA, BM 8/81, Remploy Limited, *Managing Director Report No. 250* (March 1975).
85. TNA, BM 8/49, Remploy Limited, *Minutes of the Three Hundred and Twenty-Fifth Meeting of the Board of Directors* (19 December 1974).
86. TNA, BM 8/81, Remploy Limited, *Personnel Director's Report No. 248* (January 1975); TNA BM 3/47, Remploy Limited, *Report of a Mentally Disabled Teach-In* (3 January 1975).
87. TNA, BM 8/49, Remploy Limited, *Minutes of the Three Hundred and Twenty-Fifth Meeting of the Board of Directors* (19 December 1974).
88. Ibid.
89. TNA, BM 10/48, Remploy Limited, *Report of the Working Party on 'Objectives' & Criteria of Success* (Hailey Report) (July 1980).
90. Ibid., 26.
91. Ibid., 46.
92. Ibid., 28.
93. TNA, BM 3/70, Remploy Limited, *Report of the Working Party on the Mix of Disabilities Employed by Remploy* (March 1981).
94. Ibid.
95. Ibid.
96. Ibid.
97. Ibid.
98. Ibid.

CHAPTER 7

Autism in the Twentieth Century: An Evolution of a Controversial Condition

Michelle O'Reilly, Jessica Nina Lester and Nikki Kiyimba

Introduction

Clinically, autism spectrum disorder (henceforth, autism) has been described as a lifelong neurodevelopmental condition characterised by impairments in social interaction, communication, and rigidity in thinking. Additionally, autistic individuals are typically characterised as having executive functioning difficulties (i.e. self-regulation skills), sensory processing problems (i.e. the brain processing information from the senses), difficulties with sleep and food, limited theory of mind (i.e. the ability to see things from the point of view of others), and the possibility of various co-morbid mental health conditions.[1] Despite such descriptions,

M. O'Reilly (✉)
The Greenwood Institute, University of Leicester, Leicester, UK
e-mail: Mjo14@le.ac.uk

J. N. Lester
Indiana University, Bloomington, IN, USA
e-mail: jnlester@indiana.edu

N. Kiyimba
University of Chester, Chester, UK
e-mail: n.kiyimba@chester.ac.uk

S. J. Taylor and A. Brumby (eds.), *Healthy Minds in the Twentieth Century*, Mental Health in Historical Perspective,
https://doi.org/10.1007/978-3-030-27275-3_7

autism, as we now know it, is a relatively new condition. In less than a century, a whirlwind of ideas, movements, and positions have littered the autism literature, with a critical polemic threaded through the narratives of various autistic individuals, political advocates, writers, and academic scholars. Indeed, autism is a by-product of many (even conflicting) disciplinary knowledges, institutional discourses, and histories.[2]

The twentieth century was a significant and powerful century for autism, and for some, it has been classified and understood as a '*twentieth-century disorder*'.[3] Not only were there clinical advances in terms of it being recognised, labelled, and identified and appearing in the classification systems for mental illness, but there was also the rise of pharmacology for treatment and the increased role of psychiatry for identifying and managing autism. Importantly, the twentieth century also saw a rise of critical rhetoric, challenges, political ideologies, and a range of movements, such as anti-psychiatry, critical psychiatry, neurodiversity, consumerism, and social models of disability. All these movements and perspectives made visible a struggle to invent, reconfigure, and reinvent the meaning of autism, with some challenging the position of autism as a mental health difficulty, that is, a psychiatric disability. Indeed, even in the historical present, the classification of autism as a mental health condition is controversial and contested. Later in the twentieth century, autism became redefined as a spectrum, which served to acknowledge the great heterogeneity within the meaning of autism and developed more refined ideas around the so-called impairments associated with it.

In this chapter, we overview some of the historical changes and, in doing so, highlight some challenges of labels and language that shroud those who are named autistic and/or take up this identity label. We also note the shifts in thinking that have challenged the psychiatric and psychological framing of autism. The residue of the twentieth-century tensions that is the genetic revolution, the diagnostic medicalisation, and the empowerment of neurodiversity has spilled over into the twenty-first century, leaving us with an array of critical discourses and challenges around what many now describe as a *spectrum* condition. That is, we are left with a patchwork of different perspectives and ideas regarding what constitutes autism, the language of autism, how autism should be researched, and the most appropriate healthcare pathways and other service provisions for those diagnosed. This chapter explores how this fractured view of one 'mental health difficulty' came to be. In so doing, we thread through our own position, that of social constructionism, not denying the reality of the autistic community, but acknowledging differences in views and the importance of language and meaning. Indeed, we recognise that for some autism is celebrated, treated as difference, and tensions of medical notions and impairments are proposed, and yet for others, autism is seen as disabling, the diagnosis is stressful, and treatments are actively sought. The range of perspectives that grew from the twentieth century are considered throughout. We do however insert a caveat here and note that the history of autism is vast and spans multiple disciplines and fields, and thus what follows can only ever represent a snapshot of history and inevitably misses out some of the developments that occurred throughout that century and some scholarly contributions. The chapter is only ever intended as a summary.

Early History of Autism

Importantly, the concept of autism did not specifically exist prior to the 1940s, although the notion was introduced by Bleuler in his work on schizophrenia in 1911. However, it was the work of two pioneering practitioners that identified some of the core characteristics that distinguished it as a discrete concept. First, the work of Leo Kanner, following his seminal child psychiatry text in 1935, introduced the world to the condition, autism.[4] Kanner was an Austrian psychiatrist who wrote a paper describing the behaviour he had observed in eleven children. He conceptualised these characteristics as a need for sameness, aloneness, and obsessions. It was common at this time for children with these types of behaviours to be classified as schizophrenic, so Kanner's work was important for distinguishing between the two groups. However, it should be noted here that the credit given to Kanner has created some tension and criticism.[5] Second, was the work of Hans Asperger who was writing in parallel with Kanner and wrote about the characteristics of children in similar ways.[6] Asperger was a German paediatrician who observed the behaviour of four boys who he argued were showing challenges in forming friendships, displayed a general lack of empathy towards others, had clumsy movements, and had difficulties with communication. While this work became considerably influential, it did not reach the mainstream literature until after he died. It was Asperger who noted that children with this syndrome could flourish, and in some cases show signs of genius, and expressed the insight that autism may exist on a continuum.[7] It was this notion that resurfaced, as British psychiatrist Lorna Wing introduced the notion of a spectrum.[8]

Kanner and Asperger laid a foundation therefore for understanding the behaviours of these children, and Kanner particularly argued that no single factor could explain it. However, the influence of psychoanalysis was strong during this time, and therefore, there was also a powerful promotion of the idea that there were psychodynamic causes.[9] This domination of psychoanalytic theory at this time formed the basis of a culture that blamed mothers for their child's psychological problems.[10] A hugely influential theory in the 1960s, long since discredited, was that autism was associated with a certain style of parenting, with a cold and unavailable mother leading the child to shut down emotionally.[11] Bettelheim referred to this as the '*refrigerator mother*'[12] and resulted in many mothers feeling to blame for their child's condition. This has been argued to be particularly problematic, given that evidence suggests that Bettelheim faked his medical credentials.[13]

Nonetheless, there is some persistence of mother-blaming even today,[14] despite the neurodevelopmental positioning of autism[15] and despite the extensive criticism.[16] Historically it has always been women who have carried this parental burden, as they were argued to fail to conform to the idealised view of motherhood.[17] There was a shift in thinking as psychoanalytic views lost some favour, and science took over as the predominant explanatory framework, and yet the blaming rhetoric underwent a subtle shift as mothers were not blamed via their parenting skills and style, but via their genes. The genetic and medical revolution in psychiatry positioned the aetiology of autism and other mental illnesses as having a biological origin.[18] This is something we return to shortly.

Contextualising Children

An important advancement during the first half of the twentieth century that has important implications for the development of an understanding of autism was the view of children and childhood in relation to the role of psychiatry and psychology. As Steve Taylor observes in Chapter 4, a significant period of history for child mental health was the introduction of a universal education system. In Europe and North America in the late nineteenth century, there was a new formalisation of public and private education.[19] Karim reported that it was this formalisation of education that provided a platform for adults to recognise physical and mental health conditions in the young, which subsequently in the twentieth century led to the creation of sub-disciplines such as educational psychology, social care, and developmental psychology. The increase in the social surveillance of children with the advent of compulsory education indeed engendered the necessary social conditions for the creation of autism.[20] Further, developmental psychology was especially influential and is generally credited as beginning with the work of Wilhelm Preyer in 1882 and G. Stanley Hall through his introduction of the first American Journal of Child Psychology in 1891.[21] Notably, such work at the time, into the early twentieth century was heavily influenced by the notion of the 'normal' child, underpinned by psychoanalytic ideas of childhood, which was strengthened by the specialised work of Anna Freud, Melanie Klein, and Jacques Lacan, amongst others.

The field of psychiatry also recognised the relevance and importance of treating children separately from adults, and it was in 1935 that the first child psychiatry textbook was produced by Leo Kanner. This was in parallel with the US work by Douglas Thom who developed the Boston Habit Clinic designed to help parents manage their child's everyday difficulties. This was considered necessary as following the Second World War there was recognition that children too needed help with their mental health.[22] Child psychiatry therefore became a separate sub-discipline of medicine, and one that recognised that specialist attention that was developmentally appropriate was needed, with the foundation of the American Academy of Child and Adolescent Psychiatry happening in 1953.[23] By the 1960s and 1970s, therefore, specific treatments designed for children had been developed within psychiatry and psychology.[24] Furthermore, during this period, family therapy emerged and gained popularity as it viewed the child as part of a complex social system.[25] However, it was the focus on pharmacological treatments for children that raised controversy in the later part of the twentieth century and continues today.[26] Thus, by the late twentieth century, child mental health was treated as distinctive and separate by a range of health services, including psychiatry, nursing, psychology, and education. Such services for children relied on childhood being constructed as a series of stages, with a separate focus on adolescence.

Diagnosing Autism: The Introduction of Standardised Manuals

A crucial historical moment in conceptualising autism was the development of standardised manuals. We present an overview of the main diagnostic manual, the Diagnostic and Statistical Manual of Mental Disorders (DSM) to demonstrate some of the key shifts in thinking about autism. While we recognise that there was some influence of the International Classification of Diseases (ICD), this system was much broader and contained physical illness, whereas the DSM was designed specifically for mental illness. The DSM was designed so that those working in the field of mental health were able to classify the full range of mental health conditions based on standardised criteria for diagnosis.[27] In other words, the DSM defined what does and does not constitute an illness and by default implies what constitutes normality and therefore a 'healthy mind'.[28]

The development of the DSM and the role of psychiatry have to some extent influenced how 'normal' is viewed, and the American Psychiatric Association decided to unify the diagnostic processes with the creation of DSM-I. Notably, however this single manual was not published until 1952.[29] This first edition represented an important paradigmatic change about the conceptualisation of mental illness and was a milestone in the creation of diagnostic categories. This first version contrasted two core groups of conditions, those caused by organic brain dysfunction and those with aetiology in environmental circumstances.[30] The second version, DSM-II, was developed quite quickly because of concerns about inconsistencies in the first. This version had 193 diagnostic categories, was heavily influenced by psychoanalysis, and launched in 1968.[31] This version of the DSM transformed psychiatry from a field that was concerned with pathology, to one that was more concerned with the boundaries of normality.[32] During this time, the rise of psychopharmacology was influencing more biological and neurological explanations of mental illness. Consequently, the diagnostic criteria were proposed as ways to ensure that standardisation could be achieved.[33]

The notion of standardisation underpinned new changes to the system, and in the resulting DSM-III, there were substantial changes from DSM-II. DSM-III contained criteria which identified categories but moved to a multi-axial system for diagnoses,[34] and while the revision began in 1974, it was not published until 1980.[35] This version held nearly 500 pages and 265 categories.[36] The USA was especially influential here with its insurance health system, as they demanded more precise diagnostics and were more reluctant to fund long-term therapies like psychotherapy.[37] What is especially relevant to our discussion in this chapter is that it was the advent of DSM-III in 1980 that recognised autism as a distinct conceptual category, almost 40 years after its inception by Kanner.[38]

It was this point in the twentieth century, with the inclusion of autism on the DSM-III that the work of Kanner and Asperger were revived by two British professionals who coined the notion of autistic spectrum disorder[39] and the triad of impairments became part of common clinical discourse.[40] This triad consisted of three core characteristics of autism;

1. Impairments in social interaction
2. Impairments in communication
3. Restrictive repetitive patterns of behaviour.

This was later reconfigured in the twenty-first century as a dyad of impairments and reconstructed as autism spectrum disorder, but the notion of the spectrum has been maintained.

A quick succession of revisions occurred after this with DSM-III-*R*, to DSM-IV, and DSM-IV-*R* which each reflected a round of changes. Again, relevant to our discussion, is that DSM-IV saw the inclusion of Asperger's Syndrome and this was viewed as distinct to autism.[41] Those with Asperger's Syndrome were seen as having normal or higher levels of intellectual ability, and those with the diagnosis often argue that this is fundamental to their identity.[42]

DSM 5: Autism in the Twenty-First Century

DSM-5 is the first of the manuals in the twenty-first century and reflects the modern revision from DSM-IV-*R*. Notably, this version was represented with numbers rather than Roman numerals. This new version, DSM-5, has created a great deal of controversy and was created during a period of critical thinking around mental illness more generally. The development of DSM-5 began at the end of the twentieth century and unlike its predecessors was subject to public scrutiny because of the rise of the internet.[43] By 2010, the first draft was posted online and returned over 8000 comments, with 2000 further comments in 2011 on the revision.[44] By this point, the DSM had grown to 947 pages and 541 diagnostic categories.[45]

This new version of DSM had some important changes for autism. While the notion of the spectrum was maintained, other changes were more controversial. For example, this version saw the removal of Asperger's Syndrome as a distinct classification. Indeed, Asperger's Syndrome had a short shelf-life in terms of official diagnosis, as it was not formally recognised until the 1990s and was then removed in 2013, being subsumed under the general category of autism spectrum disorder. The rationale for its removal was to reflect the shift from a categorical system to a dimensional one.[46] This however has caused great unrest in the autistic community,[47] as new interest groups have emerged claiming that classifications are a blueprint for their identity and not just an arbitrary means for classifying conditions.[48]

The criteria for diagnosing autism also shifted, as there was a move away from a triad of impairments, to a dyad of impairments, as we noted earlier. Thus, there were now just two domains of difficulties—social communication and restrictive and repetitive patterns of behaviour.[49] However, Wing et al. argued that there were relevant clinical reasons why social interaction and communication were treated separately on the triad, and therefore, collapsing them into one domain was viewed as inappropriate.[50]

The shifts in diagnosis and classification from the original version in 1952 to the latest version in 2013 have shaped and impacted on the meaning of autism and the language used to describe it. Autism is a condition that has invoked a great deal of debate and controversy in terms of the language and labels used and adopted and this has not been straightforward. As Kenny et al. noted,

> Tensions surrounding the language of autism are attributable, in part, to the very different ways that autism touches people's lives; some experience it personally, others through their children and others still might only encounter autism in some aspect of their lives – at school, at work, in the community or through friends and family.[51]

The terms used and the language adopted around autism have changed over time, with a range of different conceptualisations of the condition, including, autism, autistic spectrum disorder, autism spectrum disorder, autism spectrum condition, Asperger's syndrome, pervasive developmental disorder, and high functioning autism.[52] The different labels used are loaded with category rich inferences, and these can have different meanings for different individuals and their families.

The tensions and debates within public and academic communities regarding the most appropriate ways to conceptualise autism has been a consequence of growing disquiet about the role of psychiatry and the influence of medicine, as well as the rise of critical perspective.[53] During the twentieth century, there was a shift towards person-first language when describing individuals diagnosed with autism, so that the person came first, and the disability came after, that is, person with autism.[54] Over time however, this position has changed and further controversy about descriptive language has been proposed. Disability-first language is now more generally accepted to be the most appropriate way of describing autism, that is, an autistic person. This is because disability-first language adheres to the principle of putting a positive pronoun in front of the noun and thus removes the suggestion that autism is intrinsically negative.[55] This is especially important for the autism community who often view their autism as an accepted and instrumental part of their identity.[56] A good example of this was offered by Hagan who argued that society would not describe someone who was creative as 'a person with creativity', they would be a creative person and as such treats the creativity as part of who they are.[57] Perhaps unsurprisingly then, research has shown that diagnosed individuals tend to favour the concept of 'autistic person', but interestingly professionals still favour 'person with autism'.[58]

The Genetic Revolution

An important contribution to the rise of science and medicine was advances in the study of genetics. Psychiatry and medicine advocated organic causes of mental illness, and geneticists began to seek ways to isolate the gene(s) responsible for autism. This notion of aetiology had important implications for how we view autism and for the position of autistic people in society. The geneticisation of deviance worked to provide accounts for behaviour that failed to conform to social norms and thus provided new ways of thinking about stigma.[59] In other words, those with diagnosed conditions were now constructed as less blameworthy for their condition where it had a biological origin rather than a psychosocial one.[60]

Such a turn to science has had consequences for research and funding. The field of autism research became reenergised by genetics studies. This generally increased pace in the late-1990s, when a link between two chromosomes, 15q and 7q, were identified as connected to autism.[61] Consequently, large funding streams have been provided to further the credibility of genetic explanations, so that the aetiology may be uncovered, and medical treatments created that target the core symptoms. However, it is arguably concerning that this energy has resulted in a dominance of genetics in the study of autism at the expense of other kinds of necessary and needed research. Statistics from the UK have shown that autism research is now preoccupied with biomedical issues, as 56% of studies have explored brain, biology, and condition, and a further 15% on aetiology, and only 18% on interventions, 5% on services, and 5% on diagnosis.[62] The picture is similar in the USA, which spends 18 times the amount of the UK, but again biologically grounded work receives significantly greater income than other areas.[63]

The inappropriateness of this lack of balance in research funding streams has been positioned from a range of different views. For example, some have argued that autism is an incredibly complex and heterogeneous condition, and it is unlikely that scientists will be able to isolate a single autism gene.[64] Arguably more concerning is the risk or threat perceived by the autistic community in terms of the potential for genetic testing, which may put mothers under pressure to terminate their pregnancy.[65] Waltz noted that for autism this is especially concerning as the spectrum is broad and it is likely that multiple genes are connected, and this termination potential may threaten the lives of autistic people who could be functional in society. Some scholars have extended this argument further by claiming that the genetic focus in autism research reflects a new wave of eugenics.[66]

The diversion of research resources to genetics research is also problematic for those already diagnosed as autistic. Critics and autistic advocates have argued that by prioritising genetics research, necessary finances have been diverted away from those who need support now.[67] Arguably, there is a need for more research which focuses on the agendas that matter to autistic people and their families.[68] In our own work, we found that genetics research and the notion of a cure for autism was a low priority for autistic people and their families, and what they really wanted was more work to help them manage difficult behaviour, challenging sleep patterns, coping with adversity, and improving quality of life.[69] The research base that has an impact on the lives of autistic people and their families is insufficient, and medical and genetic evidence is inconclusive or contested.[70] It seems therefore that the priorities of medical researchers and funding councils are at odds with autistic self-advocates and families.[71] In practice, this means there is a gap between our knowledge and practice, and we need to advance our research to meet the needs of those who would benefit from it most, by focusing on issues that affect people's daily lives.[72] Specifically, we argue that there is a need for much more qualitative research that promotes the need to listen to the voices of autistic people and their families and allows for an exploration and focus on their views, opinions, and experiences.

The Challenge of Anti and Critical Psychiatry

The dominance of genetics and medicine in the field of autism has caused tensions for scholars and advocates throughout the twentieth century and into the twenty-first. As the different versions of the DSM evolved and changed, and the dominance of genetics and pharmacology grew, there was a notable shift in thinking about psychiatry as a discipline, the conceptualisation of mental illness (and more specifically tensions in classifying autism that way), and the ways in which diagnosed individuals ought to be treated and embedded in society. By the mid-twentieth century, there was a great deal of tension regarding the turn to science and medicine for answers regarding mental illness, and questions were raised about the credibility of categorising illness purely in biological ways and treatment with medications. Notably, movements during this latter half of the century were the anti-psychiatry and the critical psychiatry movement, which gained momentum as new and different critical arguments emerged.

It was during the 1960s that the international anti-psychiatry movement was recognised as such, as was a term coined by David Cooper.[73] This movement was noted to be motivated by anger and the perceived arbitrariness of diagnosis.[74] Those advocating anti-psychiatry called for a paradigm shift in terms of understanding mental illness and argued that patients were being marginalised.[75] Fundamentally those taking this position opposed the use of medication, which was the main form of treatment in the field. Furthermore, they opposed the power of psychiatrists and considered the practices to be coercive (see, e.g., Foucault).[76] The mid-twentieth century therefore saw three critical periods of anti-psychiatry, as noted by Furnham:

1. The early 1950s, where there was a conflict between psychiatrists adopting psychoanalytic perspectives and those new ideas around biology.
2. The 1960s saw a range of influential figures, such as Szasz, Basaglia, Foucault, Laing, and Cooper, from within and outside of psychiatry.

3. In the 1970s and 1980s, American and European sociology joined the debate, particularly in relation to labelling ideas and stigma, and popular media began to spotlight the practices of the profession.[77]

It was thus during the 1980s that anti-psychiatry began to lose its momentum, as psychiatrists began responding to the critique, changing their practices, and working in a more biopsychosocial way. This biopsychosocial perspective of formulating and working with mental illness began to address some of those concerns about treatment of the mentally ill.[78] Thus, anti-psychiatry as a movement failed to establish itself as a mainstream ideology embraced by mental health professionals.[79] A further paradigmatic shift occurred therefore in the 1990s, with a softer critique of psychiatry emerging under a new guise of critical psychiatry.[80] The notion of critical psychiatry was coined by David Ingleby through the collection of essays into a monologue.[81] This recognised the change from focusing on the institution to the community but retained recognition of the difficulties of psychiatry and the political issues surrounding the field. This movement began to gain some acceptance, even amongst those practicing psychiatry.[82]

The focus for critical psychiatry was that psychiatry was a powerful field, and this should be moderated by the voices of service users as central to decisions made.[83] This movement thus proposed two core issues with psychiatry. First, they argued that there are challenges to the scientific basis of psychiatric classification, and second, they noted moral problems that are a consequence of diagnosis.[84] The reliance on science and the turn to genetics were viewed as fundamentally problematic, as the biological basis of mental illness was argued to be overstated as the evidence fails to offer sufficient support for this thesis.[85]

One of the core concerns in the rising movements that had varying degrees of opposition to psychiatry, particularly from those concerned with autism, was that mental illness, and in this case autism, was being over-medicalised and thus ignoring the ecological and systemic frameworks around an individual. The significantly progressive number of diagnostic categories with each version of the DSM was argued to be increasingly medicalising behaviour of individuals, reducing social expectations of normal behaviour.[86] Such an increase of conceptualisations of abnormality created by diagnostic manuals is a cause for concern, particularly in the context of autism, and the medicalisation of autism has been especially contested.

The concept of medicalisation refers to the process of human experience being reduced to medical terms and definitions.[87] It is this medical vocabulary that validates professionals' determination of what constitutes sickness, and who qualifies as being categorised as psychiatrically disabled.[88] For the critical psychiatrists, psychiatry is a discipline that medicalises the mind as a way of legitimising the requirement of medicine to manage conditions[89] and this perpetuates an illusion that medicine provides a theoretically viable view of disability, which in turn, is tied to the notion of recovery and the restoration of the healthy mind.[90] In other words, this perspective constructs the person's illness as dispositional, and those who are unable to be 'fixed' by medicine are inappropriately labelled as deficient in some way.[91] Such a goal of normalisation denies agency to those with disabilities[92] and risks judgements of laziness, weakness or belligerence.[93] By the end of the twentieth century, healthcare was seen as consumer-driven and patient-centred, and these changes increased the tension between rising medicalisation and increased resistance to it.[94] Furthermore, the DSM-5 was argued to rely more heavily on medicalisation than any of its predecessors,[95] because of lowered thresholds, which separate individuals from the optimal society.[96]

For autism, these arguments are especially pertinent. The autism diagnostic process lacks definitive measures, and while there are tools to facilitate the process, the decision relies mostly on the subjective judgement of professionals applying the criteria, and thus, the power of medicine to define, diagnose, and treat autism has come under criticism.[97] There is therefore an extensive literature that expresses dissatisfaction with the medicalisation of autism as failing to adequately meet the needs of the autistic community.[98] This has been further hindered by the medicalised notions of deficit and cure, as medicalisation has encouraged the search for a cure.[99] Through this, autism has been constructed as a biological fact[100] and the social and cultural aspects inherent to the language of autism have been given less attention.[101] Consequently, autistic people and their families are frequently renegotiating what constitutes normal behaviour and such deviations from the norm are called to account.[102]

The ambition to 'fix' disability is central to medicalised practices, and for many autistic people, this provides a perspective that they are 'broken' in some way.[103] Such ideas are co-constructed by the mental health profession and taken directly from medical, psychological, neurological, and developmental positions of autism as grounded in the criteria created through DSM-5.[104] Importantly, autistic individuals do not use the same knowledge spheres or frames of reference as professionals, and their relationships with services can be stressful and in some cases conflicting.[105]

It may seem that medicalisation as a concept is negative; yet, notably medicalisation is not inherently problematic. The view of medicalisation as being viewed as good or bad rests on the implicit definitions of health and illness and a critical perspective regarding the effectiveness of medicine to address the well-being of the individual.[106] Indeed, the founders of medicalisation theory, such as Peter Conrad, described medicalisation as value neutral.[107] Furthermore, it must be recognised that medicalisation does serve some function for patients and families. It provides a basis to legitimise concerns that may otherwise be dismissed, and although there are risks that society takes on psychiatric concepts as identity terms, access to support largely relies on medics to confirm the nature of the problems.[108] Thus, the medical hegemonic position on autism underpins a legislative requirement to access services, as without an official diagnosis and label families are not entitled to help.[109] The flip side to this, however, is that parents may fear that if they fail to follow medical advice they will be morally implicated in any later negative experience.[110]

Despite the value neutral nature of medicalisation, it has brought with it a very particular orientation to mental health; that is, one focused on 'fixing' the presumably 'broken' individual. In contrast to this, more social constructionist understandings afford nuanced and layered understandings of difference and disability. More particular to autism, there is a need to shift away from a focus on the medicalisation to language, with its overreliance on medical explanations regarding autism.[111] Such an overreliance might lead to the mismeasurement of the autistic experience.[112] Indeed, this shift has implications for whether autism might be viewed as a natural identity or a dilemma.[113] This focus on language and the social construction of disability and normal identity were encapsulated by a related movement, that of neurodiversity.

Neurodiversity: Empowering Autism

> The language that we use has the power to reflect and shape people's perceptions of autism.[114]

A core focus of the neurodiversity movement is on the language we use around autism. This movement rejects medicalised negative concepts such as 'disorder', 'deficit', and 'impairment' and instead reconstitutes autism as a way of being.[115] The neurodiversity movement therefore directly challenged framing autism in a medicalised way. The notion of neurodiversity can be traced to Australian sociologist Judy Singer and journalist Harvey Blume, and it became popular with civil rights groups in the late-1990s.[116] The popularity of neurodiversity as a movement arose mostly online in response to what was argued to be a marginalisation of autistic people.[117] Thus, this movement sought to establish a culture where autistic people could have pride in their autistic identity and provide mutual support in self-advocacy.[118]

An underpinning principle of neurodiversity was the foundational idea of a 'differently wired brain'.[119] This movement has been instrumental in advocating strength-based discourses for autism,[120] but also for other brain-related conditions.[121] For autism, neurodiversity has two main claims as outlined by Jaarsma and Welin:

1. That autism is simply a natural variation in humans, and being neuro-diverse or neurotypical, reflect different ways of being human.
2. That neurodiversity connects to human rights, political issues, and non-discrimination of autistic people.[122]

This movement therefore became associated with the struggle for civil rights for those individuals diagnosed with neurodevelopmental conditions[123] and as such became a counter-argument for the deficit model to prevent discrimination.[124] This is important, as society tends to be organised around neurotypical values and by contrast autism is positioned as a deficit.[125]

As will be seen in Chapter 8, an important aspect of neurodiversity is that the autistic community were instrumental in its promotion and development. Indeed, there are many autistic self-advocates who have celebrated autism as part of their identity and see their autism as a natural variation.[126] Some of these people have expressed fears that the seeking of a 'cure' may result in the eradication of autism.[127] It was argued therefore that by constructing autism as synonymous with impairments, it raises questions about what it means to be human, and those failing to conform to the dominant ideology are positioned as impaired.[128]

We would note here that not all those in the autistic community advocate a neuro-diverse position, and it is important to have some balance in these arguments. Some neurodiversity movement advocates have acknowledged that some aspects of autism can cause distress and their amelioration or control is sometimes useful, and they do not oppose all forms of intervention and treatment.[129] Notably, some parents of children with autism do actively pursue treatments for their child and may even seek a cure for the condition.[130] Parents of course should have the right to seek early intervention for their offspring and have the freedom to work in ways they see as best for their child.[131] For those promoting neurodiversity, there is a position of promoting well-being and adaptive functioning to support autistic people.[132] The balance therefore is to support the notion for treatment, support, and services to overcome some of the potentially disabling effects of the condition, while steering away from medicalisation, negative language of deficiency, and damaging stereotypes that reify difference.[133] Neurodiversity as a movement and the construct of an autistic disability do not have to be incongruent, as individuals may have areas of strength and celebrate their identity, while still having some difficulties.[134]

A central underpinning concern that has arisen from medicalisation and from neurodiversity therefore is the way in which autism is classified. While medicalisation advocates the appropriateness of autism as a mental health condition, as reified through its presence on the DSM, neurodiversity tempers this position, critically questioning the 'deficit' associated with such constructions. Ultimately, therefore, questions have been raised as to whether autism should be viewed by medicine, and by society more widely, as a psychiatric disability. The rise of the neurodiversity movement in the latter part of the twentieth century had a significant impact on the way we view autism and contributed greatly to this debate. The construction of autism as a psychiatric category, as a mental health condition, and as a disability is therefore dependent upon different points of view, different theoretical frameworks, subscription to different disability models, and personal experiences and viewpoints.

In our own work, we attempt to strike a balance between recognising the real distress of some families and the severity of symptoms for some children, against the critical and imperative challenges to the notion of deficit and the importance of empowering autistic people. It is important to be aware that for some families the diagnosis of autism is stressful, and the condition can have some disabling effects on the autistic person and their families.[135] For others, a more positive view of autism is necessary and the language surrounding the autistic identity is crucial in challenging deficit, stigma, and unacceptable stereotyping. Arguably, we should not see dysfunction, but we should see difference.[136]

This is a helpful perspective that has been recognised in research with autistic people and those who live or work with them. In our own research on this issue, we considered how the notion of a disability might be understood discursively in relation to autism.[137] Using focus groups with a range of stakeholders, including autistic adults, parents of autistic children, mental health practitioners, researchers, and service managers, we found that the notion of a disability is fluid, contestable, and socially constructed. For example, an autistic adult in the focus groups argued that autism is not a disability:

> I'm a great believer that ↑autism[138] itself actually isn't a disability in any way at a::ll (.) in fact there are many areas where I would argue that my autism >is a s↑trength.[139]

However, a mother of an autistic daughter, actively disagreed, noting that autism is a disability:

> I kinda disagree< because (0.6) wouldn't you say that (0.4)<some of th::e> the like from the <triage> of autism (0.2) >the symptoms< (.) ↑a::re a symptom of the condition which is autism…….So it is a disability.[140]

There was little agreement amongst participants as to whether autism constitutes a psychiatric disability as discussions permeated the boundaries of normality versus abnormality, disability versus ability, and medicalisation versus neurodiversity. While there was some acceptance that, clinically, categorisation and diagnosis were essential for support and service provision, and that some autistic people encountered more severe levels of difficulty than others, there was also an advocacy that autism was a fundamental characteristic of personhood and should not be characterised in limiting ways.

Drawing Conclusions: Our Personal View of Autism in the Twentieth Century

Our focus has predominantly been the evolution of autism throughout the twentieth century, exploring the various paradigmatic shifts that occurred and polar arguments that developed to influence our thinking around autism. However, these influences, research ideas, medical ideologies, genetic revolution, critical discourses, movements, and personal advocacies have all influenced our understanding of autism today. We now have a fractured view of a heterogeneous condition with a spectrum of characteristics, and of autistic people being different and reflecting a multitude of identities, views, opinions, and experiences. The twenty-first century is now plagued by the notion of an autism epidemic, and medicalised questions about where such an influx of autistic individuals has come from. This means that parents are thrown into a '*minefield of conflicting information*'.[141] Indeed, the volume of information is a confusing and time-consuming area for parents.[142] Yet, in some ways, this has been positioned as hope for parents, as 'the first decade of the new century was a time of hope for many families, as parents told me they felt optimistic that science was on the verge of finally unravelling the mystery of their children's condition'.[143]

Such 'hope' and challenges related to autism are important as the 'epidemic' of the twenty-first century has become part of the medical rhetoric. There are few epidemiological studies of autism, but it is generally agreed that the prevalence currently stands at approximately 1% of the population.[144] Similarly, in childhood, a total prevalence of 116.1 per 10,000 was presented.[145] Baird et al. argued that the rates of autism are now much greater than was previously seen, and yet the reasons for such an increase in incidence are unclear.[146] The consequences of this growth have meant that services are having to rapidly expand to meet the greater demands.[147] Such an increase has however been controversial, as some have argued that it reflects an exaggeration of the existence of the condition, and others claiming it reflects the broader criteria.[148] It is therefore arguably not a new scientific discovery, but a shifting cultural and social practice regarding the social construction as to what counts as normal.[149]

We conclude our chapter by presenting our perspective on this controversial issue and in so doing recognise the validity in different perspectives. In a personal and professional sense, we acknowledge our own experiences of autism. The lead author (O'Reilly) is an academic psychologist who has a brother diagnosed with autism, currently living in an institution due to the severity of his condition and the expanse of personal need. Furthermore, in addition to the academic position, O'Reilly also works as a research consultant for a Child and Adolescent Mental Health Service and therefore works alongside a multi-disciplinary team of mental health practitioners. The second author (Lester) is a former autism teacher in the USA, has a niece diagnosed with autism, and is now an academic working in educational autism research. The third author (Kiyimba) is an academic and chartered clinical psychologist, who specialises in trauma, and has worked professionally both with clients with autism, and as a clinical supervisor of mental health professionals working with autism, as well as supervising professionals who are autistic themselves. In outlining this personal position, we reflexively acknowledge that no text can ever be produced without influence and some imposition of the values and experiences of the writer, and our views and motivations are inspired and underpinned by our personal circumstances.

Thus, in our work on autism, we favour social constructionism as a guiding theoretical position, recognising the importance of language, and taking a child-centred and family-centred approach to research. We see the value of balancing the perspectives of psychiatrists, psychologists, other mental health professionals, autistic people, autistic advocates, families, and other stakeholders. The focus, for us, should be on meaning-making, that is, on the language used in different contexts and the impact that this has. In taking this social constructionist position, we do not deny the reality of autistic people or their families. This was eloquently expressed in a recent text by Thomas et al.:

> This is not to deny the reality of mental health issues within people's lives, but rather to acknowledge that if we are to comprehend the ubiquity and impact of mental distress within a contemporary UK context, then we need to recognise the ways that particular types of scientific knowledge and particular narratives of distress have been invested with meaning and authority, and as such, have the potential to become tools for use in the pursuit of broader political agendas.[150]

The twentieth century saw many changes in the scientific and medical community understanding of autism. What we understand about autism is 'constantly in flux'.[151] Autism as a condition has created much interest, amongst researchers, scientists, the public, and the media, and this is likely due to the multiplicity of meanings.[152] We have argued that autism is a social construct. In so doing, we have recognised that for some autistic people, their autism is celebrated, but for other families it is distressing, and they struggle to cope with what they frame as adversity.[153] We have woven a narrative that is congruent with the autonomy of those with lived experiences, have favoured a person-centred position, and explored alternative ways of thinking about the pervasive medicalised discourses that have constructed autism as a psychiatric disability.

We have recognised that there are economic, institutional, and social consequences of adopting different social constructions of autism.[154] Through our exploration of the different arguments, we have shown how the dominant ideas of the impaired autistic person have become reified through medical rhetoric and the genetic revolution. We argued that psychiatry and other mental health professions have an important place for autism but acknowledge that the embracing of biopsychosocial framings of autism within those fields is important. We also noted that social constructionism provides a way for easing some of the tensions and a focus on language sets autism centre stage and challenges narrow interpretations of normality. The neurodiversity movement will be considered in greater depth by Erika Dyck and Ginny Russell in Chapter 8.

Acknowledgements We are very grateful to two reviewers who provided very useful feedback on this chapter. We thank Professor Katherine Runswick-Cole, University of Sheffield (UK) and Professor Jason Lee, De Montfort University (UK).

Notes

1. Khalid Karim, Alvina Ali, and Michelle O'Reilly, *A Practical Guide to Mental Health Problems in Children with Autistic Spectrum Disorder: 'It's Not Just Their ASD!'* (London: Jessica Kingsley Publishers, 2014).
2. Majia Nadesan, *Constructing Autism: Unravelling the 'Truth' and Understanding the Social* (New York: Routledge, 2005).
3. Nadesan, *Constructing Autism*, 29.
4. Leo Kanner, "Autistic Disturbances of Affective Contact," *Nervous Child* 2 (1943): 217–250.
5. Steve Silberman, *Neuro-Tribes* (London: Allen & Unwin, 2015).
6. Hans Asperger, "*Die 'Autistischen Psychopathen' im Kindesalter* [Autistic Psychopaths in Childhood]" (in German), *Archiv für Psychiatrie und Nervenkrankheiten* 117 (1944): 76–136.
7. Silberman, *Neuro-Tribes.*
8. Lorna Wing, "Language, Social and Cognitive Impairments in Autism and Severe Mental Retardation," *Journal of Autism and Developmental Disorders* 11, no. 1 (March 1981): 31–44.
9. Khalid Karim, "The Value of Conversation Analysis: A Child Psychiatrist's Perspective," in *The Palgrave Handbook of Child Mental Health: Discourse and Conversation Studies*, eds. Michelle O'Reilly and Jessica Nina Lester (Basingstoke: Palgrave Macmillan, 2015), 25–41.

10. Michelle Lafrance and Suzanne McKenzie-Mohr, "The DSM and Its Lure of Legitimacy," *Feminism and Psychology* 23, no. 1 (February 2013): 119–140.
11. Bruno Bettelheim, *The Empty Fortress* (New York: Free Press, 1967).
12. Sometimes this is referred to as the 'icebox' mother.
13. Silberman, *Neuro-Tribes.*
14. Michelle O'Reilly and Jessica Nina Lester, *Examining Mental Health Through Social Constructionism: The Language of Mental Health* (Basingstoke: Palgrave, 2017).
15. Karim et al., *A Practical Guide to Mental Health.*
16. Linda Blum, "Mother-Blame in the Prozac Nation: Raising Kids with Invisible Disabilities," *Gender and Society* 21, no. 2 (April 2007): 202–226.
17. Debra Jackson and Judy Mannix, "Giving Voice to the Burden of Blame: A Feminist Study of Mothers' Experiences of Mother Blaming," *International Journal of Nursing Practice* 10, no. 4 (August 2004): 150–158.
18. Jo Phelan, "Genetic Bases for Mental Illness—A Cure for Stigma?" *Trends in Neurosciences* 25 (2002): 430–431.
19. Karim, "The Value of Conversation Analysis." See also: Majia Nadesan, "Constructing Autism: A Brief Genealogy," in *Autism and Representation*, ed. Mark Osteen (New York: Routledge, 2008), 78–95.
20. Ibid.
21. Joseph Rey Francisco Assumpção, Carlos Bernad, Fusun Çuhadaroğlu, Bonnie Evans et al., "History of Child and Adolescent Psychiatry," in *IACAPAP E-Textbook of Child and Adolescent Mental Health*, ed. Joseph Rey (Geneva: International Association for Child and Adolescent Psychiatry and Allied Professions, 2015).
22. Kathleen Jones, *Taming the Troublesome Child* (Harvard: Harvard University Press, 1999).
23. Rey et al., "History of Child."
24. Karim, "The Value of Conversation Analysis."
25. Rudi Dallos and Ros Draper, *An Introduction to Family Therapy: Systemic Theory and Practice* (3rd edition) (Berkshire: Open University Press, 2010).
26. Karim, "The Value of Conversation Analysis."
27. American Psychiatric Association, *Diagnostic and Statistical Manual of Mental Disorders* (5th edition) (Washington: American Psychiatric Association, 2013).
28. Karim, "The Value of Conversation Analysis."
29. George Raines, "Comment: The New Nomenclature," *American Journal of Psychiatry* 109 (1953): 548–549.

30. Shadia Kawa and James Giordano, "A Brief Historicity of the Diagnostic and Statistical Manual of Mental Disorders: Issues and Implications for the Future of Psychiatric Canon and Practice," *Philosophy, Ethics and Humanities in Medicine* 7, no. 2 (December 2012). https://doi.org/10.1186/1747-5341-7-2.
31. Edward Shorter, *A History of Psychiatry: From the Era of the Asylum to the Age of Prozac* (New York: Wiley, 1997).
32. Allan Horwitz, *Creating Mental Illness* (Chicago: University of Chicago Press, 2002).
33. Shorter, *A History of Psychiatry.*
34. Blashfield et al., "The Cycle of Classification."
35. Rick Mayes and Allan Horwitz, "DSM-III and the Revolution in the Classification of Mental Illness," *Journal of the History of the Behavioural Sciences* 41, no. 3 (Summer 2005): 249–267.
36. Shorter, *A History of Psychiatry.*
37. Ibid.
38. Fred Volkmar and Joe McPartland, "From Kanner to DSM-5: Autism as an Evolving Concept," *Annual Review Clinical Psychology* 10, no. 1 (December 2014): 193–212.
39. Lorna Wing and Judith Gould, "Severe Impairments of Social Interaction and Associated Abnormalities in Children: Epidemiology and Classification," *Journal of Autism and Developmental Disorders* 9, no. 1 (March 1979): 11–29.
40. Wing, "Language, Social and Cognitive Impairments."
41. David Giles, "'DSM-V Is Taking Away Our Identity': The Reaction of the Online Community to the Proposed Changes in the Diagnosis of Asperger's Disorder," *Health* 18, no. 2 (June 2013): 179–195.
42. Tony Attwood, *The Complete Guide to Asperger's Syndrome* (London: Jessica Kingsley Publishers, 2007).
43. Blashfield et al., "The Cycle of Classification."
44. Ibid.
45. APA, *Diagnostic and Statistical Manual.*
46. Richard Bentall, *Doctoring the Mind: Why Psychiatric Treatments Fail* (London: Allen Lane, 2009).
47. We use the term "autistic community" to refer to individuals who self-identify as autistic and/or have a diagnosis of autism.
48. Giles, "DSM-V."
49. APA, *Diagnostic and Statistical Manual.*
50. Lorna Wing, Judith Gould, and Christopher Gillberg, "Autism Spectrum Disorders in the DSM-V: Better or Worse that the DSM-IV?" *Research in Developmental Disabilities* 32, no. 2 (March 2011): 768–773.

51. Lorcan Kenny, Caroline Hattersley, Bonnie Molins et al., "Which Terms Should Be Used to Describe Autism? Perspectives from the UK Autism Community," *Autism* 20, no. 4 (May 2016): 442–462, 442.
52. Karim et al., *A Practical Guide to Mental Health.*
53. Kenny et al., "Which Terms Should Be Used?"
54. Joan Blaska, "The Power of Language: Speak and Write Using 'Person First,'" in *Perspectives of Disability*, ed. Mark Nagler (Palo Alto: Health Markets Research, 1993), 5–32.
55. Helena Halmari, "Political Correctness, Euphemism, and Language Change: The Case of 'People First'," *Journal of Pragmatics* 43, no. 3 (February 2011): 828–840. See also: John Robison, *Be Different: Adventures of a Free-Range Aspergian with Practical Advice for Aspergians, Misfits, Families and Teachers* (New York: Crown Publishing Group, 2011).
56. Joyce Davidson and Victoria Henderson, "'Coming Out' on the Spectrum: Autism, Identity and Disclosure," *Social and Cultural Geography* 11, no. 2 (March 2010): 155–170.
57. Karen Hagan, *Discourses in Autism Assessment and Diagnosis* (Unpublished PhD thesis, The Open University, Milton Keynes, 2018).
58. Kenny et al., "Which Terms Should Be Used?"
59. Jo Phelan, "Geneticization of Deviant Behaviour and Consequences for Stigma: The Case of Mental Illness," *Journal of Health and Social Behaviour* 46, no. 4 (2005): 307–322.
60. Sheila Mehta and Amerigo Farina, "Is Being 'Sick' Really Better? Effect of the Disease View of Mental Disorder on Stigma," *Journal of Social and Clinical Psychology* 16, no. 4 (1997): 405–419.
61. Carolyn Schanen, "Epigenetics of Autism Spectrum Disorders," *Human Mol Genetics* 15, no. 2 (2006): 138–150.
62. Elizabeth Pellicano, Adam Dinsmore, and Tony Charman, *A Future Made Together: Shaping Autism Research in the UK* (Centre for Research in Autism and Education Institute of Education, University of London, 2013).
63. Pellicano et al., *A Future Made Together.*
64. Rebecca Muhle, Stephanie Trentacoste, and Isabelle Rapin, "The Genetics of Autism," *Paediatrics* 113 (2004): 472–486.
65. Mitzi Waltz, "Autism=Death: The Social and Medical Impact of a Catastrophic Medical Model of Autistic Spectrum Disorders," *Popular Narrative Media* 1, no. 1 (2008): 13–24.
66. Michael Orsini and Joyce Davidson, "Introduction: Critical Autism Studies, Notes on an Emerging Field," in *Worlds of Autism: Across the Spectrum of Neurological Difference*, eds. Joyce Davidson and Michael Orsini (Minneapolis: University of Minnesota Press, 2013), 1–30.

67. Elizabeth Pellicano and Mark Stears, "Bridging Autism, Science, and Society: Moving Toward an Ethically Informed Approach to Autism Research," *Autism Research* 4, no. 4 (August 2011): 271–282.
68. Pellicano et al., *A Future Made Together.*
69. Michelle O'Reilly, Khalid Karim, and Jessica Nina Lester, "Should Autism Be Classified as a Mental Illness/Disability? Evidence from Empirical Work," in *The Palgrave Handbook of Child Mental Health; Discourse and Conversation Studies*, eds. Michelle O'Reilly and Jessica Nina Lester, (Basingstoke: Palgrave Macmillan, 2015), 252–271.
70. Sami Timimi, J. Gardner, and B. McCabe, *The Myth of Autism* (London: Palgrave Macmillan, 2010).
71. Pellicano et al., "Bridging Autism."
72. Pellicano et al., *A Future Made Together.*
73. David Cooper, *Psychiatry and Anti-psychiatry* (London: Tavistock Publications, 1967).
74. Michael Staub, *Madness Is Civilization* (Chicago: University of Chicago Press, 2011).
75. Oliver Ralley, "The Rise of Anti-psychiatry: A Historical Review," *History of Medicine Online* (November 2012).
76. Michel Foucault, *History of Madness* (trans. J. Murphy and J. Khalfa) (London: Routledge, 2006).
77. Adrian Furnham, "Anti-psychiatry Movement: It Is 55 Years Since the Myth of Mental Illness: What Was That All About?" (2015). https://www.psychologytoday.com/blog/sideways-view/201505/the-anti-psychiatry-movement. Accessed 15 February 2016.
78. David Rissmiller and Joshua Rissmiller, "Evolution of the Anti-psychiatry Movement into Mental Health Consumerism," *Psychiatric Services* 57, no. 6 (June 2006): 863–866.
79. John Hopton, "The Future of Critical Psychiatry," *Critical Social Policy* 26, no. 1 (February 2006): 57–73.
80. Rob Whitley, "The Anti-psychiatry Movement: Dead, Diminishing, or Developing?" *Psychiatric Services* 63, no. 10 (October 2012): 1039–1041.
81. David Ingleby, ed., "Understanding 'Mental Illness'," in *The Politics of Mental Health* (Harmondsworth: Penguin, 1981), 23–71.
82. Phillip Thomas, "What Is Critical Psychiatry?" (2013). http://www.madinamerica.com/2013/01/what-is-critical-psychiatry/. Accessed 13 December 2016.
83. Phillip Thomas and Patrick Bracken, "Critical Psychiatry in Practice," *Advances in Psychiatric Treatment* 10, no. 5 (September 2004): 361–370.
84. Phillip Thomas, "What Is Critical Psychiatry?"
85. Duncan Double, "The Limits of Psychiatry," *British Medical Journal* 324, no. 13 (April 2002): 900–904.

86. Til Wykes and Felicity Callard, "Diagnosis, Diagnosis, Diagnosis: Towards DSM-5," *Journal of Mental Health* 19, no. 4 (August 2010): 301–304.
87. Peter Conrad and Kristin Barker, "The Social Construction of Illness: Key Insights and Policy Implications," *Journal of Health and Social Behaviour* 51, S (2010): s67–s79.
88. Sarah Nettleton, *The Sociology of Health and Illness* (3rd edition) (Cambridge: Polity Press, 2013).
89. Thomas Szasz, "Psychiatry, Anti-psychiatry, Critical Psychiatry: What Do These Terms Mean?" *Philosophy, Psychiatry, & Psychology* 17, no. 3 (January 2010): 229–232.
90. Jan Grue, "Discourse Analysis and Disability: Some Topics and Issues," *Discourse and Society* 22, no. 5 (August 2011): 532–546.
91. Stephen Gilson and Elizabeth DePoy, "Child Mental Health: A Discourse Community," in *The Palgrave Handbook of Child Mental Health: Discourse and Conversation Studies*, eds. Michelle O'Reilly and Jessica Nina Lester (Basingstoke: Palgrave Macmillan, 2015), 117–138.
92. Gil Eyal et al., *The Autism Matrix: The Social Origins of the Autism Epidemic* (Cambridge: Polity Press, 2010).
93. LaFrance and McKenzie-Mohr, "The DSM and Its Lure of Legitimacy."
94. Karen Ballard and Mary Ann Elston, "Medicalisation: A Multi-dimensional Concept," *Social Theory and Health* 3, no. 3 (July 2005): 228–241.
95. Tom Strong, "Brief Therapy and the DSM: 13 Possible Conversational Tensions," *Journal of Brief Therapy* 9, nos. 1–2 (2014): 1–12.
96. Allen Frances, *Saving Normal: An Insider's Revolt Against Out-of-Control Psychiatric Diagnosis, DSM-5, Big Pharma, and the Medicalization of Ordinary Life* (New York: William Morrow, 2013).
97. Karim et al., *A Practical Guide to Mental Health.*
98. Steven Kapp et al., "Deficit, Difference, or Both? Autism and Neurodiversity," *Developmental Psychology* 49, no. 1 (January 2013): 59–71. See also: Russell Razzaque and Lisa Wood, "Open Dialogue and Its Relevance to the NHS: Opinions of NHS Staff and Service Users," *Community Mental Health Journal* 51, no. 8 (November 2015): 931–938.
99. Alicia Broderick and Ari Ne'eman, "Autism as Metaphor: Narrative and Counter Narrative," *International Journal of Inclusive Education* 12, nos. 5–6 (September 2008): 459–476.
100. Ruth Glynne-Owen, "Early Intervention and Autism: The Impact of Positivism and the Call for Change," *International Journal of Children's Rights* 18, no. 3 (January 2010): 405–416.

101. Majia Nadesan, *Constructing Autism: Unravelling the 'Truth' and Understanding the Social* (New York: Routledge, 2005).
102. Jessica Nina Lester and Trena Paulus, "'That Teacher Takes Everything Badly': Discursively Reframing Non-normative Behaviours in Therapy Sessions," *International Journal of Qualitative Studies in Education* 27, no. 5 (2014): 641–666.
103. Mark Osteen, ed., "Autism and Representation: A Comprehensive Introduction," in *Autism and Representation* (New York: Routledge, 2008), 1–47.
104. Hagan, *Discourses in Autism.*
105. Nick Hodge and Katherine Runswick-Cole, "Problematising Parent-Professional Partnerships in Education," *Disability and Society* 23, no. 6 (October 2008): 637–647.
106. Dorothy Broom and Roslyn Woodward, "Medicalisation Reconsidered: Toward a Collaborative Approach to Care," *Sociology of Health and Illness* 18, no. 3 (1996): 357–378.
107. Erik Parens, "On Good and Bad Forms of Medicalization," *Bioethics* 27, no. 1 (January 2013): 28–35.
108. O'Reilly and Lester, *Examining Mental Health.*
109. Kristin Bumiller, "Quirky Citizens: Autism and the Anti-normalization of Politics," *Annual Meeting of the American Political Science* 33, no. 4 (June 2008): 967–991.
110. Juanne Clarke and Gudrun van Amerom, "'Surplus Suffering': Differences Between Organizational Understandings of Asperger's Syndrome and Those People Who Claim the 'Disorder'," *Disability and Society* 22, no. 7 (November 2007): 761–776.
111. Olga Solomon, "Body in Autism: A View from Social Interaction," in *Language, Body and Health*, eds. Paul McPherron and Vaidehi Ramanathan (Berlin, Germany: Walter de Gruyter, 2011), 105–144.
112. Nick Chown, "The Mismeasure of Autism: A Challenge to Orthodox Autism Theory," *Autonomy, the Critical Journal of Interdisciplinary Autism Studies* 1, no. 2 (May 2013): 1–10.
113. Jessica Nina Lester, Khalid Karim, and Michelle O'Reilly, "Autism Itself Actually Isn't a Disability: The Ideological Dilemmas of Negotiating a 'Normal' Versus 'Abnormal' Autistic Identity," *Communication & Medicine* 11, no. 2 (November 2015): 139–152.
114. Kenny et al., "Which Terms Should Be Used?"
115. Ibid.
116. Thomas Armstrong, *Neurodiversity: Discovering the Extraordinary Gifts of Autism, ADHD, Dyslexia, and Other Brain Differences* (Cambridge: Da Capo, 2016). See also: Nobuo Masataka, "Implications of the Idea of Neurodiversity for Understanding the Origins of Developmental Disorders," *Physics of Life Reviews* 20 (November 2016): 85–108.

117. Francisco Ortega, "The Cerebral Subject and the Challenge of Neurodiversity," *BioSocieties* 4, no. 4 (December 2009): 25–445.
118. Dana Baker, *The Politics of Neurodiversity: Why Public Policy Matters* (Boulder: Lynne Rienner, 2011).
119. Ortega, "The Cerebral Subject."
120. Pier Jaarsma and Stellan Welin, "Autism as a Natural Human Variation: Reflections on the Claims of the Neurodiversity Movement," *Health Care Analysis* 20, no. 1 (March 2012): 20–30.
121. Michael Orsini, "Autism, Neurodiversity and the Welfare State: The Challenges of Accommodating Neurological Difference," *Canadian Journal of Political Science* 45, no. 4 (December 2012): 805–827.
122. Jaarsma and Welin, "Autism as a Natural Human Variation."
123. Andrew Fenton and Timothy Krahn, "Autism, Neurodiversity and Equality Beyond the 'Normal'," *Journal of Ethics in Mental Health* 2, no. 2 (November 2007): 1–6.
124. Katherine Runswick-Cole, "'Us' and 'Them': The Limits and Possibilities of a 'Politics of Neurodiversity' in Neoliberal Times," *Disability & Society* 29, no. 7 (May 2014): 1117–1129.
125. Charlotte Brownlow, "Presenting the Self: Negotiating a Label of Autism," *Journal of Intellectual and Developmental Disability* 35, no. 1 (March 2010): 14–21.
126. Baker, *The Politics of Neurodiversity*; Kapp et al., "Deficit, Difference, or Both?"
127. Pellicano and Stears, "Bridging Autism."
128. Waltz, "Autism=Death."
129. Ari Ne'eman, "The Future (and the Past) of Autism Advocacy, or Why the ASA's Magazine, *The Advocate* Wouldn't Publish This Piece," *Disability Studies Quarterly* 30, no. 1 (February 2010). See also: Runswick-Cole, "'Us' and 'Them'."
130. Brigitte Chamak, "Autism and Social Movements: French Parents' Associations and International Autistic Individuals' Organizations," *Sociology of Health and Illness* 30, no. 1 (2008): 76–96.
131. Simon Baron-Cohen, "Editorial Perspective: Neurodiversity—A Revolutionary Concept for Autism and Psychiatry," *Journal of Child Psychology and Psychiatry* 58, no. 6 (May 2017): 744–747.
132. Kapp et al., "Deficit, Difference, or Both?"
133. Orsini, "Autism, Neurodiversity."
134. Baron-Cohen, "Editorial Perspective."
135. Jaci Huws and Robert Jones, "Diagnosis, Disclosure, and Having Autism: An Interpretative Phenomenological Analysis of the Perceptions of Young People with Autism," *Journal of Intellectual and Developmental Disability* 33, no. 2 (2008): 99–107.

136. Meng-Chuan Lai et al., "Subgrouping the Autism 'Spectrum': Reflections on DSM-5," *PLoS Biology* 11, no. 4 (April 2013): e1001544.
137. Lester et al., "Autism Itself Actually Isn't a Disability."
138. The symbols in these quotations of data are from the Jefferson CA system.
139. Ibid., 143.
140. Ibid., 144.
141. Silberman, *Neuro-Tribes*, 13.
142. Michelle O'Reilly, Khalid Karim, and Jessica Nina Lester, "Separating 'Emotion' from 'the Science': Exploring the Perceived Value of Information for Parents and Families of Children with ASD," *Clinical Child Psychology and Psychiatry* 20, no. 3 (April 2015): 500–514.
143. Silberman, *Neuro-Tribes*, 12.
144. Traloch Brugha et al., *Autism Spectrum Disorders in Adults Living in Households Throughout England: Report from the Adult Psychiatric Morbidity Survey 2007* (The NHS Information Centre for Health and Social Care, 2009).
145. Gillian Baird, Emily Simonoff, Andrew Pickles, et al., "Prevalence of Disorders of the Autism Spectrum in a Population Cohort of Children in South Thames: The Special Needs and Autism Project (SNAP)," *Lancet* 368, no. 9531 (2006): 210–215.
146. Ibid.
147. Karim et al., *A Practical Guide to Mental Health.*
148. Eyal et al., *The Autism Matrix*; Sami Timimi, "Autism Is Not a Scientifically Valid or Clinically Useful Diagnosis," *British Medical Journal* 343 (August 2011): d5105; Wykes and Callard, "Diagnosis, Diagnosis, Diagnosis."
149. Timimi et al., *The Myth of Autism.*
150. Felicity Thomas et al., "Moral Narratives and Mental Health: Rethinking Understandings of Distress and Healthcare Support in Contexts of Austerity and Welfare Reform," *Palgrave Communications* 4, no. 39 (April 2018): 2.
151. Kenny et al., "Which Terms Should Be Used?"
152. Orsini and Davidson, "Critical Autism Studies."
153. Hodge and Runswick-Cole, "Problematising Parent-professional Partnerships."
154. Jessica Nina Lester and Michelle O'Reilly, "Repositioning Disability in the Discourse of Our Times: A Study of the Everyday Lives of Children with Autism," in *Education, Equity, and Economy*, eds. George Noblit and William Pink (London: Springer, 2016), 133–160.

CHAPTER 8

Challenging Psychiatric Classification: Healthy Autistic Diversity the Neurodiversity Movement

Erika Dyck and Ginny Russell

Introduction

Beginning after the Second World War, amid the momentum of civil rights, feminism and gay and lesbian rights movements, patients' rights groups began campaigning for their place in the human rights discourse. Disability rights activists engaged in aggressive campaigns for better access to services, while psychiatric patients and their families began lobbying for anti-stigma campaigns, alongside demands for adequate housing, basic health services, voting rights, and access to safe employment. The concept of 'mad pride' emerged in the 1960s and, like other pride movements, challenged the notion that madness, or gayness,

E. Dyck
Department of History, University of Saskatchewan,
Saskatoon, SK, Canada
e-mail: erika.dyck@usask.ca

G. Russell (✉)
University of Exeter, Exeter, UK
e-mail: G.Russell@exeter.ac.uk

S. J. Taylor and A. Brumby (eds.), *Healthy Minds in the Twentieth Century*, Mental Health in Historical Perspective,
https://doi.org/10.1007/978-3-030-27275-3_8

or femaleness, was a disease to be treated rather than an identity to be celebrated.[1] At its heart, mad pride campaigns took aim at psychiatry for codifying mental health into a system of deficits and disorders that required medical interventions to fix, rather than look to political action as a mechanism for producing a culture of acceptance. The late twentieth century has been a time of expansion in both the utilisation of the diagnostic label of autism and the reach of the 'neurodiversity' concept, and we situate the work of this group in the context of previous patient movements.

Embracing 'madness' as a preferred term over ones such as mental disease, defect, disability, or illness reconnected an experience with an identity that was not necessarily the product of a medical encounter. Intellectuals in the 1960s began critiquing modern social values, in part, by analysing the history psychiatry and how it had evolved into a form of policing behaviour. They held psychiatry accountable for passing judgement on human value and in harnessing their practice to a political system that equated human worth with productivity.[2] Classifications systems, such as the Diagnostic and Statistical Manual of Mental Disorders (DSM), they argued, merely institutionalised a practice of pathologising undesirable or unproductive people.

Famously, French philosopher, Michel Foucault in his first book *Folie de la Raison* (1961), translated into English under the title, *Madness and Civilization* (1965), trenchantly critiqued the rise of psychiatry and how it psychiatrised and attempted to control normal behaviour.[3] Madness, for Foucault, not only existed as a state that predated the rise of psychiatry as a discipline, but was also reminiscent of a point in time when mad people had a small degree of autonomy and when madness itself was part of one's character, not an affliction, label, or burden. Foucault lamented the rise of a modern world where psychiatrists wielded significant and, in his view, illegitimate power to determine what was and what was not acceptable behaviour. In a society where free will was leached away by modern aspirations of productivity, capital accumulation, and moral authority, Foucault critiqued how this world order created opportunities for individuals to police normalcy and to discipline members of society. His influential work on this topic ricocheted through the intellectual community and contributed to the rise of anti-psychiatry during the 1960s.

Some contemporary critics, including Thomas Szasz, a psychiatrist ultimately based in California, pronounced that 'mental illness was a myth', which had no basis in scientific or medical reasoning.[4]

The evolution of an 'anti-psychiatry' perspective, which sometimes cross-fertilised with post-modernism, provided fodder for critiques of psychiatry and its institutions. Another 1960s critical scholar, Erving Goffman, focused his doctoral work specifically on the way in which the institution itself produced abnormal behaviours, due to the disciplined existence within its walls, the rhythms of institutional life, and the reinforced labels that one was forced to adopt while 'playing a role' or meeting the expectations of a psychiatric diagnosis.[5] Scottish psychiatrist R. D. Laing added further grist to the mill by provocatively suggesting that madness offered insights into higher orders of consciousness; in other words, madness stimulated creativity, intelligence and allowed an individual to see past certainties held in check by the majority of society—the so-called sane.[6]

These academic critiques provided some of the intellectual, philosophical, and linguistic foundations for a more widespread social movement, which was populated by individuals who had consumed and survived mental health services (henceforth referred to as consumer/survivor movements). The timing was important. In the 1960s, governments throughout North America and Europe began closing, downsizing, and repurposing large psychiatric hospitals. Thousands of patients were moved into communities, unleashing a new host of challenges as former patients carried stigmatising labels, behaviours, and habits with them into communities that were often unwelcoming.[7] This major transition in mental health service provision—from asylum-based care to an undifferentiated matrix of health, welfare, education, and labour support—also gave rise to new forms of activism, as former patients and their families repositioned themselves in civil society.

Mad pride, the disability rights movement, the recovery movement, and other consumer/survivor movements emerged alongside these intellectual critiques of psychiatry and provided a poignant example of people denouncing psychiatric labelling and instead turning psychiatric experiences into sources of insight, authority, and expertise. The rise of consumer/survivor movements that ensued can be considered as a form of 'biosociality' a term coined more recently by Rabinow to describe common health identities linked by social networks.[8] What the new movements seem to share is a repudiation of 'victim' status and a push towards greater equality with those who are considered experts, clinicians, researchers, or professionals who become involved after diagnosis. They demanded a greater involvement in determining research priorities and policy decisions.[9] Thanks in part to these groups, the power and credibility of their first-person voice—the voice of affected individuals—are increasingly acknowledged nowadays in health policy and clinical guidelines.

The 1960s patients' rights movements that relied on anti-psychiatry critiques have evolved considerably and have splintered and developed different approaches under the umbrella of social health activism. Today, one area of resistance to psychiatric labelling channelled by patients themselves is from those who have been diagnosed with neurodevelopmental conditions of childhood such as attention deficit hyperactivity disorder, dyslexia, Tourette's syndrome, and in particular autism. A politically mobilised group of adults with autism spectrum disorder (here referred to as ASD or simply autism), and sometimes their relatives, pioneered the neurodiversity movement (NDM). The NDM voice rejects society's disablement of difference while advocating a neurological/medical model for autistic behaviour. In this chapter, we examine the position of the NDM, with reference to other mental health consumer/survivor/patient movements and their challenges to psychiatric classification in the past.

The Neurodiversity Movement

> I am autistic. I've always been autistic, and I always will be autistic. Autism is part of who I am, just as my sense of humor and my emotions are part of me. I like who I am, even my autistic part.[10]

'Neurodiversity' is a concept that implies that neurological difference is best understood as an inherent and valuable part of the range of human variation, rather than a pathological form of difference. The NDM met and mobilised in the late twentieth century through utilising websites such as *Aspies for Freedom, The Autist, Autcom, Angelfire, Wrongplanet, and Neurodiversity.com,* most of which are based in the USA or Europe. Numerous online chat rooms, blogs, and fora are springing up where autistic adults discuss common interests and make friends across international and geographical boundaries. The rise of the internet in the late twentieth century enabled mobilisation and creation of online communities in geographically dispersed areas, occupying virtual social spaces that are constructed and normative in their effects.[11] Many autistic people started 'coming out' with pride, asserting minority cultural status, adopting similar strategies to the earlier gay rights movement. Many of the arguments of the NDM relate to the autism diagnosis as a category or label. NDM voices taken from open access neurodiversity and autism sites are quoted here to illustrate their position.

The theory of labelling has a long history and activists and practitioners alike have struggled to come to terms with whether psychiatric labels help to reduce stigma and encourage research and treatment, or whether they merely reinforce a particular negative characterisation of behaviour that becomes a self-fulfilling prophecy. The neurodiversity movement in this respect is not unlike other survivor, consumer, or disability rights campaigns that both resist labels and rely on labels to forge a sense of community. Even amongst the most radical anti-psychiatry groups, the relationship with medical language has produced a common touchstone for identifying community and fostering a more positive image of identity. For example, Canada's earliest expression of organised mad pride emerged in the 1960s from a consortium of people who had been institutionalised for psychiatric disorders in Vancouver. As they discussed the appropriate name for their community-based group, they settled on Mad Patients' Association (MPA). The name blended philosophies of the de- or anti-medicalised term 'madness' with the explicit term 'patient', conveying a relationship with medicine. This self-conscious choice of names thus embraced the ethos of the survivors, or the radical edge of anti-psychiatric views—those who survived in spite of psychiatric interventions, and the consumer model—those who have relied on psychiatric services, from the perspective of an autonomous client or user.

Autism as a Diagnostic Category

Kanner and Asperger first described 'insistence on sameness' and 'autistic aloneness' over 70 years ago.[12] As was explained by O'Reilly, Lester, and Kiyimba in Chapter 7, according to today's DSM-5, autism diagnosis is given where there is (1) impairment in behaviours within the social/communication domain and (2) sensory issues and/or repetitive behaviours. Autism as a phenotype thus creates a category of persons who share social/communication impairment and repetitive behaviours, although the evidence that these symptoms are co-inherited is fairly weak.[13] Essentially, the diagnosis depends on a deficit-based description of a person, creating a 'spoiled identity' in Goffman's terms. Since the first epidemiological prevalence estimates were conducted in the 1970s the autism diagnosis has seen an exponential rise, changing from a diagnosis given to an estimated one in two thousand to one in forty children. This rise is partly due to increased awareness and partly due to changing boundaries of diagnostic criteria, with intellectually able individuals included in the category of Asperger's disorder in the 1990s. Such changes, coupled with the advent of the internet, meant that for the first time, many twentieth-century children were identified with autism, and as they grew up, many had the means, the motivation, and the intellectual resources to challenge a purely medical understanding of ASD. In the 1990s, Martijn Dekker of the Netherlands founded Independent Living on the Autistic Spectrum (InLv), an e-mail list for autistic people. First run by hand on dial-up, InLv was the first fully autistic-run, self-hosted online autism community. The effect was to promote discussion of how autism could be a benefit as well as create challenges, fostering in its subscribers a 'healthy autistic' identity. The community became the forerunner to the NDM.

Autism is not currently identified by neurological markers as none are reliable enough to create diagnostic tests, although ASDs are classified as 'neurodevelopmental disorders' in the DSM. Despite the NDM's focus on the 'neuro', it is behavioural inventories that are used to diagnose ASD, not brain scans, and these use a dimensional scale of impairment with a cut-off rather than a dichotomous distinction. In the diagnostic process, the point at which individual differences in behaviour constitute autism is based on clinical decisions which may depend on resources that diagnosis will trigger, the meaning of diagnosis to the patient or clinicians' own ideas about signs and signifiers of autism. This, a somewhat arbitrary cut-off is used on the autism spectrum to define autism as a diagnosed disorder. This process is heavily influenced by culture, context, and values.[14] Chloe Silverman argues that the concept of autism as a diagnostic category has been established in the DSM and International Classification of Disease (ICD) and stabilised through the work of institutions such as schools, gene banks, professional associations, charities, government committees, parent networks, and those with vested interest in treatments.[15] The DSM and ICD systems are tools for classification of disorder that are themselves shaped by moral and historical values.[16] These aspects underscore the shifting nature of autism diagnosis and remind us that the idea of ASD as a fixed underlying biological/neurological entity (the purely medical model) requires qualification. Moreover, part of the pushback on these categories is coming from people who have been placed in them.

The Position of the NDM

The NDM has articulated a number of central features or core values, all of which stem from a denial of pathologisation and a critique of labelling as a harmful action against diversity. Each of these tenets is discussed below:

Opposing Elimination and Cure
Opposition to Cure of autism was frequently expressed as a rationale for online activity of NDM members:

> We are deeply concerned with the perception of autism as a disorder and the attempts to cure and prevent autism. In addition we are concerned about attempts to help autistic people that actually harm them. The purpose of this website is to educate the public about the anti-cure perspective.[17]

Michelle Dawson, a Canadian academic diagnosed with autism, has questioned the ethics of treatments such as applied behaviour analysis (ABA) and appeared as an expert witness in the 2004 legal case where parents of autistic children filed to get medical insurance to cover the cost of treatment, claiming it was a medical necessity. Her position was that ABA's techniques of aversion, which persistently expose children with ASD to stimuli that cause distress and subsequently discourage unwanted behaviours such as hand-flapping, are tantamount to cruelty. Dawson considers these unwanted behaviours to be coping mechanisms in stressful situations:

> Where ABA needs scrutiny is when its power is used to remove odd behaviours which may be useful and necessary to the autistic (such as rocking, flapping, and analytical, rather than social or 'imaginative' play); and when typical, expected behaviours which may be stressful, painful, or useless to the autistic (such as pointing, joint attention, appropriate gaze, and eye contact) are imposed.[18]

Others within the movement have criticised therapies, which attempt to remove autistic behaviours, claiming for example that the repetitive behaviours are valid attempts to communicate.[19]

> Neurotypical people pity autistics. I pity neurotypicals. I pity anyone who cannot feel the way that flapping your hands just so amplifies everything you feel and thrusts it up into the air. ... A boy pacing by himself, flapping and humming and laughing. ...A shake of the fingers in front of the eyes,

> a monologue, an echolaliated phrase. All of these things autistic people are supposed to be ashamed of and stop doing? They are how we communicate our joy.[20]

In their opposition to 'elimination' and invoking the term 'genocide', the NDM has drawn on and shares a stance with the earlier 'survivor' movement. Similarly, people who were sexually sterilised under the eugenics programme in Alberta, Canada, have worked closely with community advocates and scholars to produce a 'survivor'-based website that examines the history of eugenics from their perspectives.[21] Survivors reject psychiatry outright, likening psychiatric treatment to a form of slavery and an outright abuse of power. Anthropologist Gabriella Coleman has suggested that some people have embraced that language of survival—much akin to the language of the NDM—strategically to underscore their resilience after decades, even centuries, of oppression.[22] The resulting movement, Coleman contends, 'mobilizes the cultural ideal of freedom and self-determination, along with the law of human rights and informed consent, to undermine the moral, scientific, and legal claims furthered by the pharmaceutical companies and other authoritative psychiatric institutions'.[23] Survivors represent the most radical voices within mad culture, connecting their survival, self-consciously, to a form of resilience. This terminology intentionally invites connotations of genocide by linking identity with a social group, such as a race or ethnicity.[24]

Use of Neurocentric/Medical Models

The NDM seems to have its roots in the social model of disability, which separates physical and biological impairment from the disabling attitudes and practices of society.[25]

> People with autistic spectrum disorders are not victims of autism, they are victims of society. They do not suffer from their developmental differences, they suffer from prejudice, ignorance, lack of understanding, exploitation, verbal abuse - all this and more from that sector of society which considers itself socially able.[26]

The NDM has also sprung from the twentieth-century trend dubbed 'neurocentrism' by Satel and Lilienfeld who define neurocentrism as 'the view that human experience and behavior can be best explained from the predominant or even exclusive perspective of the brain', which they argue, has increasingly been adopted in parallel with the rise of neuroscience throughout the last half of the last century and into this.[27] Applying neurological explanations to one's mind has further been described by Rose as the 'neurochemical self'.[28] Neurocentrism is therefore a description of the extent to which neuroscientific theories, practices, technologies, and therapies are influencing how we view ourselves (those identities and characteristics ascribed to self and views of others). The term 'neurodiversity' implies the movement predominantly understand their differences in terms of innate neurology, the brain and/or wiring, perhaps underpinned with genetic causes. Language has been developed describing people as either 'neurotypical' (NT, not on the autism spectrum) or 'neurodivergent', i.e. people like themselves (non-NT). 'Neurotypical' is a term now widely adopted in academic neuroscience. The NDM, then, uses the language of brain wiring or neurology to explain the nature of their differences. The differences in how the brain communicates then result in behavioural differences. One NDM advocate explained it this way:

> Another common sign that someone is an NT? Touching. NTs enjoy all sorts of physical contact and often use touch to greet friends, family and even casual acquaintances... NTs are simply wired differently.[29]

As the autism phenotype is well-established, research coalesces around it. Neuroscientific research charts uniformities and abnormalities in the brain that make it possible to distinguish an autistic brain from a normal brain. Neuroscience seeks tangible, discrete differences between autistic and non-autistic brains while epidemiology tells us ASD is a spectrum condition extending into the sub-clinical range. In this way, neuroscience researchers tend to dichotomise brain structure for what is essentially a dimensional condition. By looking at differences between dichotomised autistic/non-autistic phenotypes (as opposed to a dimensional spectrum of traits in the whole population), medical neuroscience models tend to homogenise autistic brains.[30] This is analogous to the dichotomisation of difference between 'neurotypical' and 'neurodivergent' persons identified by the NDM; it refers to an essential difference in brain structure and/or functioning. Thus, the NDM adopts a position that both challenges and shores up medicalisation: while questioning autism and other neurodevelopmental conditions as diagnosable 'disorders', it utilises a model derived from neuroscientific research.

The rise of neurocentrism is transdisciplinary in its reach. Historian Daniel Smail has developed this idea as an overarching ontology that, if applied carefully, has the potential to disrupt our commonly held beliefs about diversity and difference over time. He proposes a 'neuro-historical' approach that locates the beginning of history at a moment when humans approach a state of consciousness; he defines this moment in neuro-biological terms as the evolutionary stage that separates humans from animals. Pinpointing this moment, he argues, requires careful collaboration with scientists to sift through new kinds of evidence—biological and neurochemical evidence—to re-interpret the origins of history. Part of Smail's justification for a turn to neuro-history is that it offers a deeper, richer account of humanity by acknowledging human bio[neuro]-diversity. He recommends shifting the historians' gaze away from political structures, social arrangements, or even cultural expressions and looking instead to neuro-history.[31] This conceptualisation of neurodiversity is not unlike some of R. D. Laing's suggestions in the 1960s that schizophrenia could be productively understood as an alternative form of consciousness. Rather than view psychotic symptoms as deficits or abnormal characteristics, Laing considered that delusions, paranoid ideation, and other kinds of behaviour might produce a form of intelligible insight into human interactions.[32]

Objections to Diagnosis as a Category of Disorder

Diagnosis of autism is recommended by health guidelines as an essential way to access treatments.[33] However, many autistic adults in the NDM feel that both experts and families misinterpret or take no notice of them.[34] Autism, they argue, should not be considered as pathological, i.e. in terms of a medical condition, but in terms of the normal variation of the human population; thus, many in their ranks oppose medical description in terms of diagnosis of an ASD.

> The autistic community firmly believes that autism is not a disorder but a natural human variation. We are deeply concerned with the perception of autism as a disorder.[35]

A core argument is that the extreme end of the autism spectrum (i.e. reaching diagnostic thresholds) is required for the existence of a healthy gene pool in the human population. Without these people, the range of natural human variation is reduced, and the strengths that autism brings, such as ability to focus and systemising skills, will be lost. Such variation in the gene pool is desirable for evolutionary reasons, the NDM contest.

> It may be that autistic people are essentially different from "normal" people, and it is precisely those differences that make them invaluable to the ongoing evolution of the human race.[36]

This argument matches some of the historical anti-psychiatry arguments, particularly those of Laing, who suggested that people with psychotic disorders had a lot to offer society due to the gift of insight that they had into situations that non-psychotic people could not even appreciate. Within the neurodiversity movement, a similar sentiment circulates, suggesting that some autistic people also have particular areas of strength or talent formerly known in the medical literature as 'islets of ability'.[37] Members of the NDM point out that all these aspects of autism will be lost if people like them are 'cured' or aborted as babies.

> Many of the traits I identify with most strongly are those labelled autistic, such as the ability to hyperfocus, a strong attention to detail, the ability to enjoy my own company for long periods, not being controlled by the social collective, etc.[38]

There are several historical precedents where conditions have been de-medicalised in the past, through activism of politically mobilised social movements. The classic example of de-medicalisation in the twentieth century is homosexuality, which was listed as a disorder in the second edition of the DSM, becoming a treatable medical condition rather than a behaviour that had previously been seen as morally wrong. Hormone treatments and castrations were used to 'cure' homosexuality and in some cases admission to mental institutions.[39] While people were unsuccessfully 'treated' or punished for homosexual behaviour in the past, medicine now recognises it as a dimension of a normal and healthy life, thanks to sustained pressure from gay activists who mobilised around the diagnosis in the mid-century period.[40]

Parallels to the NDM objection to ASD as a devastating childhood disorder can be seen in the transgender movement's attempts to demedicalise gender identity disorder (GID) of childhood in the late twentieth century. Bryant and Burke describe in depth the opposition of the transgender movement (TGM) to this diagnostic category which first appeared in DSM-III in 1980.[41] The main objections to GID diagnosis were that sex-stereotyped behaviour was used to define children as healthy or pathological, which reinforced the binary model of gender. The TGM objected that GIDs could result in stigmatisation of transgender individuals that gender variance was no longer described as a range of valid ways to be, but rather had been redefined as a serious form of illness. The movement drew attention to treatments that were designed to intervene and 'cure' individuals of their problem. A technical objection was that existing research and clinical evidence were based overwhelmingly on study and treatment of boys, an argument that has parallels with discussions about gender and autism.[42] Overall, the TGM raised similar objections to those of the NDM today.

Like the NDM, the TGM were vocal protesters and mobilised around the diagnostic category. After a concerted writing campaign to the American Psychiatric Association (APA, authors of DSM) in 1977, concerns and correspondence led to modifications in DSM-IV, where a less behavioural-based medical definition of GIDs was adopted. GIDs in DSM-IV were also subject to sustained activist objection. By the mid-1990s, several political US-based transgender groups, including Gender Pac, National Centre for Lesbian Rights, and National Gay and Lesbian Task Force, issued stinging statements critiquing GID. In 1996, activists repeatedly picketed the APA and formed the 'National Coalition for GID Reform', and finally in 2013, GID was dropped in the DSM-5 revised diagnostic criteria. The condition was replaced with a new category 'Gender Dysphoria' which only pathologises the discontent experienced as a result of gender identity issues. Some in TGM accept the new DSM-5 definition does go some way to demedicalise GIDs and helps to resolve some of their issues. Fraser, Karasic, Meyer, and Wylie, for example, argue that changes to DSM were a direct consequence of activism and have led to a more acceptable diagnosis/ label and a reframing of the condition as they see it.[43] One parallel NDM argument is that the term 'disorder' implies a pathological state, with negative and stigmatising connotations. Autism researchers have therefore called for the term 'autism spectrum disorder' to be replaced by 'autism spectrum condition', reminiscent of the replacement of the term 'retardation' with 'learning disabilities' in the 1970s.[44] This replacement of terms and continual refinement of diagnostic criteria is an important feature of the history of psychiatric disorders. However, as Jan Walmsley explained in Chapter 5, replacing terms does not always alter stigma indefinitely.

The new term may become stigmatised as its connotation may become the same as the old term. Even replacing autism with 'neurodivergent' is simply replacing one label with another.

Embracing Labels: Being or Having?

The NDM see autism as an integral part of their identity that they are disinclined to change. The autistic activist Jim Sinclair presented a talk called 'Don't Mourn for Us' at the 1993 International Conference on Autism in Canada, addressed primarily to parents. It drew interest through its challenge to the then-dominant 'autism as tragedy' narrative, describing autism as inseparable from the person, rather than a separate disease entity, and as a valid way of being. Following this influential paper and in contrast to the requirements in medical journals, the NDM often prefer first-person language 'autistic person' to 'person with autism' as the latter implies the autism can be divorced from the individual.

> Autism is not something that I have, it is something that I am. Autism is not a cage, with us as the prisoners.[45]

Many parents, by contrast, prefer the more medical term 'person with autism'. Kit Weintraub, a parent who is a board member of Families for Early Autism Treatment, states:

> My children are not autistic, they 'have autism'.... Autism, according to the vast majority of medical experts today, causes severely abnormal development, and without appropriate treatment it can condemn those affected to a life of isolation and dependency. "Autistics" is a rather new politically-correct term that I find troubling; it is a label that attempts to define people with autism as members of an elite group of human beings who differ from the rest of us only in terms of their unique talents and their superior way of experiencing the world.[46]

However, some autistic people have argued against this viewpoint. Michelle Dawson retorted that 'person with autism' was equivalent to describing herself as a 'person with femaleness'.

> Autism is a way of being. It is pervasive; it colors every experience, every sensation, perception, thought, emotion, and encounter, every aspect of existence. It is not possible to separate the autism from the person.[47]

Examining some of the online sources suggests that that parents, teachers, and even siblings are indeed present within the NDM community, but their relationship to the movement is different. Unlike the bold statements about *being* autistic, not *having* autism—parents fill a different role in their relationship to children who are considered autistic. This triangulating effect may force us to return to a different set of historical trends. That of familiar arguments about pre-natal screening, mother-blaming, food additives, and other environmental factors that cast the net over a much wider set of influences for contributing—whether positively or negatively—to the neurodiversity identity. American philosopher and psychiatrist Carl Elliot has described this cascading effect in terms of contagion or that of being 'sick by association' or courtesy stigma idea.[48] The resulting labelling of entire families or perhaps groups creates another layer of complexity as we examine the process of identity building and forms of activism that are created to challenge or embrace these labels.

For the NDM, although opposed to the notion that they suffer from 'disorder', the label of 'autism' has become both an identity and a rallying cry. Increasingly activism occurs online, and occasionally this becomes a physical meeting. In 1995, *Autreat* was founded. This is an annual conference that accommodates autistic difficulties, e.g. participants wear colour-coded badges indicating whether or not they may be approached for conversation. *Autreat* endeavours to create an ideal NDM environment that eliminates disablement through tolerance and adaptation and challenges the status of autism as a psychiatric disorder.

Diverse Perspectives Within Social Health and Survivor Movements

As the scholarship on this topic has illustrated, the approaches taken by social health and survivor movements are varied, complex, and change over time. The language of survival versus consumption provides one broad set of generalisations for understanding the political stances within this multifaceted set of movements. Even within organised campaigns, however, there is significant granularity that can range from libertarian to socialist perspectives regarding how people should be cared for, accepted, and tolerated in modern society. Within debates over the medicalisation and treatment of addiction, for example, scholars and practitioners continue to disagree on whether the twelve-step model of recovery developed in the twentieth century offers a sufficiently de-medicalised approach, or whether it should be used at all. Some have suggested that individuals need a menu of treatment options that might change over time, which superficially may appear as though they subscribe to different models of addiction altogether.[49] The fluidity, however, is important in these rights-based campaigns as individuals develop different relationships with practitioners, services, and gaps in the mental health system.

Similarly, the position of the autistic community vis a vis diagnosis of autism is not homogenous. While some activists argue that the diagnosis of autism spectrum 'disorder' implies a pathological state, with negative and stigmatising connotations, many other adults describe their relief and understanding once a diagnosis is given; a label that makes sense of a lifetime of struggle. High profile cases have included Susan Boyle who described her relief at getting an Asperger's diagnosis, which for her, provided an explanation of her difficulties, and deflected attributions of responsibility for previous aberrant behaviour.[50] Thus, the diagnosis can have a positive effect, whereas undiagnosed, a person may have been blamed as lazy or socially tactless: diagnosis may lead to attribution of behavioural difficulties to biomedical causes, which improves others' reactions.[51]

Autism is highly heterogeneous, and individuals may range from severely intellectually impaired and/or non-verbal to 'high functioning' and articulate. Detractors of the NDM argue the online self-advocates represent only the high-functioning extreme. Indeed it may be the medicalisation of less severe autism behaviours that has ironically given impetus to the NDM, as less severely impaired individuals have rallied under the autism banner, where previously they may not have been diagnosed. Francisco Ortega, describes the movement as a form of aggressive identity politics who appropriate the right to speak on behalf of every autistic person.[52] It is certainly true that not all adults diagnosed with autism see their condition as a positive part of themselves, and some are pro-cure.[53]

> The possibility that I could be very autistic for the rest of my life always upsets me. Therefore, when people talk about a cure I actually love to hear it. To be realistic, I know I will never be cured. The cause of my autism is a genetic anomaly and can't be changed.[54]

Whether or not total de-medicalisation of autism is a desirable outcome, there are powerful forces at work that oppose this. The fact that autism is such a well-recognised phenotype with invested research, clinical and commercial worlds reliant on its existence as a medical category adds to the entrenchment of the category. Cooper describes this process and argues this makes major de-medicalisation by DSM unlikely.[55] This uncomfortable relationship with medical terminology, treatment, and a simultaneous rejection of a disordered identity is a familiar tenet of many of the social health movements and illustrates some of the inherent tensions within these campaigns.

Conclusions

The NDM movement is an example of the kind of authentic expression that attempts to take mental health and disability conditions out from clinician's control. It both uses and challenges the medicalisation of brain and behaviour in a way that offers a coherent and consistent critique of psychiatry while allowing for diversity within its members. Broderick and Ne'eman argue that the bulk of the support for framing autism within a disorder model, where it is viewed as a 'disease' external to the person comes from within the non-autistic 'NT' community, whereas the bulk of the support for framing autism within a neurodiversity model comes from within the NDM and autistic community.[56] They argue that NDM provides a counter-narrative that can play a vital role in the resistance to ideological hegemony (which they view as the medical model of autism diagnosis). They position the NDM are essentially activists in the process of de-medicalisation of autism.

However, we have found that instead of providing a homogenous oppositional set of ideas, the NDM have struggled to define their relationship with psychiatric categories much like other consumer campaigns that adopt aspects of the medical model, while rejecting wholesale psychiatric classification. Far from being a standardised voice, the NDM is also typical of other social health movement in the complex identity politics that co-mingle with the psychiatric labels, those of gender, age, sexuality, race, class amongst others, which continue to condition individual experiences.

The early phase of mad pride movement in the 1960s relied on a more homogenous notion of madness to anchor its resistance from institutionalisation and opposition to psychiatry borrowing strategies from the left, namely collective action, and from the right, especially elements of libertarianism. As the movement evolves, however, as with other social movements, identity politics have grown more complicated. The NDM provides an illustrative example of how some of those struggles have played out in a particular manifestation of experiences, ones brought together through a degree of commonality. Digital media technology, used very effectively by the NDM, also demonstrates a new layer in the discourse on consumer networks as unlike the 1960s where people needed to physically gather to generate a common set of political goals, and the internet allows for virtual meeting spaces and virtual identities.[57] It helps to complicate boundaries of citizenship and identity and offers, perhaps, a new model for consumer-survivor activism for the twenty-first century.

Acknowledgements The second author's work was generously funded by the Wellcome Trust, grant number 108676/Z/15/Z.

Notes

1. We believe the first mad pride march took place in Vancouver, Canada in 1963. It was a very small event, so small that organisers barely remember it taking place. But small though it was, it helped to put madness on the map in terms of human rights movements in the 1960s. See, "*The Inmates Are Running the Asylum*," youtube.com (2013).
2. For example, see Michel Foucault, *Madness and Civilization: A History of Insanity in the Age of Reason* (New York: Vintage Books, 1965).
3. Ibid.
4. Thomas Szasz, *The Myth of Mental Illness: Foundations of a Theory of Personal Conduct* (New York: HarperCollins, 1974).
5. Erving Goffman, *Asylums: Essays on the Social Situation of Mental Patients and Other Inmates* (New York: Anchor Books, 1961).
6. Ronald D. Laing, *The Politics of Experience and the Bird of Paradise* (London: Penguin Books, 1967).
7. For more on this topic, see Kathleen Kendall, "From Closed Ranks to Open Doors: Elaine and John Cummings' Mental Health Education Experiment in 1950s Saskatchewan," *Histoire Sociale* 44, no. 88 (November 2011): 257–286; C. Dooley, "The End of the Asylum (Town): Community Responses to the Depopulation and Closure of the Saskatchewan Hospital, Weyburn," *Histoire Sociale* 44, no. 88 (November 2011): 331–354; Gerald Grob, *From Asylum to Community:*

Mental Health Policy in Modern America (Princeton: Princeton University Press, 1991).

8. Paul Rabinow, *Artificiality and Enlightenment: From Sociobiology to Biosociality: Anthropologies of Modernity* (London: Blackwell, 1996), 91–111.
9. Vololona Rabeharisoa et al., "Evidence-Based Activism: Patients' Organisations, Users and Activist's Groups in Knowledge," *BioSocieties* 9, no. 2 (2014): 111–128.
10. "Two Autistic People Speak," *Autism News Science and Opinion*, posted December 19, 2006. https://leftbrainrightbrain.co.uk/2006/12/19/two-autistic-people-speak/. Accessed 17 March 2018.
11. Joyce Davidson, "Autistic Culture Online: Virtual Communication and Cultural Expression on the Spectrum," *Social and Cultural Geography* 9, no. 7 (November 2008): 791–806.
12. Lyons Fitzgerald, "Asperger (1906–1980) and Kanner (1894–1981), the Two Pioneers of Autism," *Journal of Autism Developmental Disorders* 37, no. 10 (November 2007): 2022–2023.
13. Francesca Happé, Angelica Ronald, and Robert Plomin, "Time to Give Up on a Single Explanation for Autism," *Nature Neuroscience* 9, no. 10 (October 2006): 18–20.
14. Courtenay F. Norbury and Alison Sparks, "Difference or Disorder? Cultural Issues in Understanding Neurodevelopmental Disorders," *Developmental Psychology* 49, no. 1 (January 2013): 45–58.
15. Chloe Silverman, *Understanding Autism: Parents, Doctors, and the History of a Disorder* (Princeton: Princeton University Press, 2011), 354.
16. Richard P. Bentall, *Madness Explained: Psychosis and Human Nature* (London: Penguin Books, 2004), 656.
17. "Autism: Pro-existance, Anti-cure." http://www.angelfire.com/space2/autism/. Accessed 17 March 2018.
18. Michelle Dawson, "The Misbehaviour of Behaviorists: Ethical Challenges to the Autism-ABA Industry" (2004). http://www.sentex.net/~nexus23/naa_aba.html, Accessed 17 March 2018.
19. A. Baggs, "In My Language" (2007) [Cited 2014 October 10]. http://www.youtube.com/watch?v=JnylM1hI2jc.
20. "The Obsessive Joy of Autism." https://juststimming.wordpress.com/2011/04/05/the-obsessive-joy-of-autism/. Accessed on 19 March 2018.
21. www.eugenics.archive.ca. Accessed 17 March 2018.
22. Gabriella Coleman, "The Politics of Rationality: Psychiatric Survivors' Challenge to Psychiatry," in *Tactical Biopolitics*, eds. Kavita Philip and Beatriz da Costa (Cambridge: MIT Press, 2008), 341.
23. Ibid.

24. For further examples of survivor documents and scholarship, see the Psychiatric Survivor Archives of Toronto; Bonnie Burstow and Don Weitz, eds., *Shrink Resistant: The Struggle Against Psychiatry in Canada* (Vancouver: New Star Books, 1998).
25. V. Finkelstein, *Changing Attitudes and Disabled People: Issues for Discussion* (World Rehabilitation Fund, 1979); Michael Oliver, *The Politics of Disablement: A Sociological Approach* (London: Palgrave Macmillan, 1997), 152.
26. Grace Hewson, "Letters to the Editor," *The Guardian* (2001) reposted on "Autism: The Question of Cure," neurodiversity.com. http://neurodiversity.com/cure.html. Accessed 17 March 2018.
27. Sally Satel and Scott O. Lilienfeld, *Brainwashed: The Seductive Appeal of Mindless Neuroscience* (New York: Basic Civitas Books, 2013), 288.
28. Nikolas Rose, *The Politics of Life Itself: Biomedicine, Power, and Subjectivity in the Twenty-First Century* (Princeton: Princeton University Press, 2006).
29. "What Is Neurotypical?" (2013). https://musingsofanaspie.com/2013/01/10/what-is-neurotypical/. Accessed 17 March 2018.
30. F. Ortega, "The Cerebral Subject and the Challenge of Neurodiversity," *BioSocieties* 4, no. 4 (2009): 425–445.
31. Daniel Smail, *On Deep History and the Brain* (Berkeley: University of California Press, 2007).
32. Laing, *Politics of Experience*.
33. Committee on Children with Disabilities, "The Pediatrician's Role in the Diagnosis and Management of Autistic Spectrum Disorder in Children," *Pediatrics* 107, no. 5 (May 2001): 1221–1226.
34. Sara O'Neil, "The Meaning of Autism: Beyond Disorder," *Disability and Society* 23, no. 7 (2008): 787–799.
35. "Autism: Pro-existance, Anti-cure." http://www.angelfire.com/space2/autism/. Accessed 17 March 2018.
36. Donna Rosinski, "Wading into the Gene Pool: Questions and Answers About Autism and Genetics." http://neurodiversity.com/cure.html. Accessed 17 March 2018.
37. Amitta Shah and Uta Frith, "An Islet of Ability in Autistic Children: A Research Note," *Journal of Child Psychology and Psychiatry* 24, no. 4 (October 1983): 613–620.
38. Elmindreda, "Don't Touch My Brain." http://neurodiversity.com/positive.html. Accessed 17 March 2018.
39. Graham Hart and Kaye Wellings, "Sexual Behaviour and Its Medicalisation: in Sickness and in Health," *British Medical Journal* 13, no. 324 (7342) (April 2002): 896–900.

40. See, for example, Gary Kinsman, "'Character Weaknesses' and 'Fruit Machines': Towards an Analysis of the Anti-homosexual Security Campaign in the Canadian Civil Service," *Labour/Le Travail* 35 (1995): 133–161; Elise Chenier, *Strangers in Our Midst: Sexual Deviancy in Post-war Ontario* (Toronto: University of Toronto Press, 2008). For contemporary controversy on this topic and psychiatrist Robert Spitzer, see, for example, Paul Harris "Psychiatrist Who Championed 'Gay' Cure Admits He Was Wrong," *The Guardian*, 9 May 2012 [Cited 10 October 2014]. http://www.theguardian.com/world/2012/may/19/psychiatrist-admits-gay-cure-study-flawed.
41. Karl Bryant, "Diagnosis and Medicalization," in *Sociology of Diagnosis*, eds. P. J. Mcgann et al. (Bingley, UK: Emerald Group Publishing, 2011); M. C. Burke, "Resisting Pathology: GID and the Contested Terrain of Diagnosis in the Transgender Rights Movement," *Sociology of Diagnosis*: 156–183.
42. Keely Cheslack-Postava and Rebecca Jordan-Young, "Autism Spectrum Disorders: Toward a Gendered Embodiment Model," *Social Science and Medicine* 74, no. 11 (July 2011): 1667–1674.
43. Lin Fraser et al., "Recommendations for Revision of the DSM Diagnosis of Gender Identity Disorder in Adults," *International Journal on Transgenderism* 12, no. 2 (2010): 80–85.
44. Simon Baron-Cohen et al., "Prevalence of Autism-Spectrum Conditions: UK School-Based Population Study," *British Journal of Psychiatry* 194, no. 6 (June 2009): 500–509.
45. "Cure for Autism?" originally from http://within.autistics.org/nocure.html, http://neurodiversity.com/cure.html. Accessed 17 March 2018.
46. Kit Weintraub, "Guest Voice: A Mother's Perspective" (2004). http://www.sentex.net/~nexus23/301-350.html. Accessed March 2018.
47. Jim Sinclair, "Don't Mourn for Us" (1993), based on an article published in the Autism Network International Newsletter, *Our Voice* 1, no. 3. http://www.autreat.com/dont_mourn.html. Accessed 17 March 2018.
48. Carl Elliot, "A New Way of Being Mad," *Atlantic Monthly* 286 (2000): 76–86.
49. See the recent debates on hamspro@googlegroups.com, in particular the tense discussions between Stanton Peele and Gabor Mate as they consider the consequences of being pigeon-holed into particular political camps within this treatment and empowerment framework.
50. Catherine Deveney, "Susan Boyle: My Relief at Discovering That I have Asperger's," *The Guardian*, 8 December 2013. https://www.theguardian.com/music/2013/dec/08/susan-boyle-autism. Accessed 17 March 2018.

51. Ginny Russell and Brahm Norwich, "Dilemmas, Dilemmas and Destigmatization: Parental Perspectives on the Diagnosis of Autism Spectrum Disorders," *Clinical Child Psychology and Psychiatry* 17, no. 2 (April 2012): 229–45.
52. F. Oretga, "The Cerebral Subject and the Challenge of Neurodiversity," *Biosocieties* 4, no. 4 (2009): 425–445.
53. Charlotte Brownlow, "Presenting the Self: Negotiating a Label of Autism," *Journal of Intellectual Development and Disability* 35, no. 1 (March 2010): 14–21.
54. Sue Rubin, "Acceptance Versus Cure" (2005). CNN.com. Accessed 17 March 2018.
55. Rachel Cooper, *Classifying Madness: A Philosophical Examination of the Diagnostic and Statistical Manual of Mental Disorders* (Dordrecht, Netherlands: Springer Science & Business Media, 2005): 198.
56. Alicia Broderick and Ari Ne'eman, "Autism as Metaphor: Narrative and Counter-Narrative," *International Journal of Inclusive Education* 12, nos. 5–6 (September–November 2008): 459–476.
57. For more on the role of the internet on this topic, see Elliott, "A New Way to Be Mad."

CHAPTER 9

The National Schizophrenia Fellowship: Charity, Caregiving and Strategies of Coping, 1960–1980

Alice Brumby

Introduction

In 1970, the newly formed Schizophrenia Action Committee claimed that 'Schizophrenia is one of the greatest crippling scourges of mankind.'[1] The pamphlet was a call to arms, seeking members to join and bolster this new organisation. It called for those with personal experience and first-hand knowledge of the condition to make themselves known and come together with like-minded people, to help and be helped in return. Schizophrenia is still in the 'unmentionable classes' of stigmatised illnesses, the pamphlet argued, highlighting that 'to drag the horrible problem into the full light of day and publicity was the only way of dealing with it.'[2] Explaining that the community care programme and new drugs meant that more schizophrenic persons were being pushed out of closing mental hospitals and back into the homes of the often unprepared and ill-equipped, good-will of families and caregivers, the article

A. Brumby (✉)
York St John University, York, UK
e-mail: a.brumby@yorksj.ac.uk

S. J. Taylor and A. Brumby (eds.), *Healthy Minds in the Twentieth Century*, Mental Health in Historical Perspective,
https://doi.org/10.1007/978-3-030-27275-3_9

concluded; 'If you agree that a new voluntary society is required, will you help?'[3]

The path to community care and evaluating the effectiveness of community care services has been widely documented by historians over the past few decades.[4] Within this history, the role of individual patients and their families has also received much attention.[5] Alex Mold has identified that historically there has been 'a culture of paternalism' within the medical profession, which advocated patients taking a largely passive role in their relationship with their doctors.[6] However, as Ali Haggett explains, 'during the 1960s, this situation began to change, heralded by the growth of post-war social surveys and the emergence of early patient advocacy groups, which demonstrated that patients wanted more information about health and disease.'[7] This emergence of early patient advocacy groups corresponds with the work of Dyck and Russell in Chapter 8 of this volume. Following on from their work however, this chapter suggests that it was not only the patients, but the families who wanted more information in the 1960s. As such, this chapter aims to recount the narrative of a collection of families who came together to form a pressure group to support each other in their quest to provide better care to their loved ones who had being diagnosed with schizophrenia.

Historically, the role of the families themselves in trying to understand their relatives' mental health condition has been well documented.[8] Historians have revealed how families were instrumental in all aspects of institutional life, from committal, to corresponding with loved ones and superintendents during treatment, to reclaiming their loved ones from the grasp of the asylum when they were in a better social or financial position to cope with their illnesses.[9] Nicole Baur has identified that patients' families could very often be extremely vocal in the recovery process for their loved ones suggesting that in the 1930s, 'many patients and relatives welcomed the new treatments, as they often provided the only glimpse of hope for a cure.'[10] By the 1960s, this relationship between families and medical authorities remained in friction, and families complained of having to deal with the 'obfuscating fog of hospital vagueness and evasiveness.'[11] One contemporary article, published in 1972, argued that 'relatives seldom have the chance to share what little they have learnt with professional workers. Still less of course, are they in the position to make themselves heard by central policy makers and social services. They are unorganised [and] shy of publicity.'[12]

Charitable bodies were not new to the mental health sector in the second half of the twentieth century. The Mental After-Care Association, established in 1879, as 'The After-Care Association for Poor and Friendless Female Convalescents on Leaving Asylums for the Insane,' was the first association to assist those recovering from mental disorder.[13] Moreover, the National Association for Mental Health [N.A.M.H] had been in existence since 1946, merging from a variety of pre-existing charities: the Central Association for Mental Welfare (founded 1913), the National Council for Mental Hygiene (established 1922) and the Child Guidance Council (formed 1927).[14] However, the evidence suggests that some families and caregivers felt unsupported by such a large and impersonal umbrella organisations.[15] Letters identified that some family members wanted more personal support groups to aid them with their individual problems and illnesses.[16] From the backdrop of these frustrations, a number of charities, pressure groups and support groups sprang up in the 1970s. The N.A.M.H itself was rebranded to become MIND in 1972, to overcome a public perception that it was becoming old-fashioned.[17]

Using the National Schizophrenia Fellowship (NSF) as a case study, this chapter will identify how different stakeholder groups, including families and caregivers, attempted to respond to government policies and the perceived shortfalls in state provision for mental health care in the late twentieth century. The origins of the NSF lay as a fellowship for those who knew, looked after, or cared for relatives, family members or friends suffering from schizophrenia. In his work, Peter Barham has described the early days of the NSF as an organisation which 'maintained an intransigently patronising attitude towards its constituents.'[18] Despite this assessment, this chapter will show that this opinion may have been created because this organisation was substantially more than just a charity for those who were suffering from schizophrenia. Instead, it was a support group, a network where the 'healthy' non-schizophrenic relative, friend or caregiver could access the support that they needed, not necessarily to care for their loved one or charge, but also to care for their own mental health needs.

This chapter will look at the beginning of the movement for a care regime and support network in the UK from the perspective of one of the very founding members of the organisation, E.A., using oral history to bring the narrative to life. Interspersed with the oral history, this chapter will also look at surviving documents from the NSF archives, looking at papers, council minutes and publications of the NSF itself. This chapter will show how the National Schizophrenia Fellowship helped to support relatives struggling with stigma and acted as a barrier to this stigma, thus providing strategies of coping for the 'healthy mind' of the non-schizophrenic caregiver. One of the arguments that are central to this chapter is that stigma manifested itself in a variety of ways. Many of the relatives and friends of those suffering from schizophrenia felt the stigma themselves, and certainly, their loved ones felt it keenly.[19] My interviewee, E.A., although proud and fiercely independent, asked to be anonymised in this chapter. The reason that was stated for desiring such anonymity is that although her brother passed away many years ago, he never wanted E.A. to talk about his 'episodes' or his times in hospital, a request that she dutifully promised. In the interview, she states, 'And so that's my anxiety now that I might let P.A. down by telling anybody.'[20] To preserve her promise to her brother and therefore to preserve his anonymity, E.A. herself must remain anonymous in this chapter. Those who may be able to identify her are asked to respect her wishes and preserve her (and therefore her brother's) anonymity.[21]

In 2002, the National Schizophrenia Fellowship underwent a rebrand to encompass a broader diversity of mental illnesses, renaming itself 'Rethink' in the process. Although as a charity, it is still registered under the name National Schizophrenia Fellowship, 'Rethink' became known as Rethink Mental Illness in 2011, officially trading under this name. Throughout the interview, E.A. uses the term 'Rethink' to refer, anachronistically, to the National Schizophrenia Fellowship. Whilst I have preserved her use of the name 'Rethink' when quoting from her interview, I have tried to preserve the appropriate historically accurate name in the text.

On Our Own, with the Medical Authorities

Like many people with schizophrenia, P.A. was in his early twenties when his symptoms first started to manifest themselves. P.A. lived with his mother and sister, in London in the mid-1960s. His father had died in the war when P.A. was just a small boy. P.A. himself had served briefly in the army and had a good service; however, by the end of his service, his problems started to become apparent. After coming out of the army, P.A. suffered a couple of suicidal attacks. In the early 1960s, before receiving diagnosis or treatment, his psychotic symptoms really started to become problematic. E.A.'s narrative identifies the struggle to receive a diagnosis and the attitudes her family experienced by both the community and medical professionals at the time.

Although, as will become clear, E.A. was evidently upset about the reaction from her neighbours, relatives and lay community more generally, the interview identifies that she felt extremely supported by the medical professionals. Within the interview, she praises the 'dear old metropolitan police,'[22] the doctors and the mental hospital that her brother was sent to and has special praise for the community psychiatric nurses [CPNs] who cared for her brother on numerous occasions throughout his illness. Nevertheless, at the outset of her brother's illness, E.A. identifies how receiving a diagnosis by any medical professional proved challenging. E.A. recounts how at the beginning of the illness, in the early 1960s, when P.A. had just started to become 'very psychotic' every attempt to achieve a diagnosis was hindered:

> But every time this GP made an appointment for P.A., P.A. said that there was nothing wrong. We told P.A. that he had to let the doctor look at him, but every time the GP came, he said there's nothing wrong, there's nothing wrong with me and that's why it went on such a long time, before he could get treatment. So we never actually managed to get him the appointment that he needed.[23]

P.A.'s first treatment in a mental hospital was eventually secured in 1964. His route to treatment began during one of P.A.'s psychotic attacks. After aimlessly wandering for hours one January night without a coat, P.A. was confronted by the police, and he ended up in a Magistrates' Court for hitting a policeman.[24] After this, he was remanded in custody for the night and the following day:

> The magistrate recommended that he go to Brixton Prison hospital for assessment by a medical person, for about four weeks [...] The prison medical officer wrote to mum and he said in his opinion he had observed that P.A. was in the early stages of paranoid schizophrenia, which if left untreated could lead to certification [...] He said that he intended to recommend to the magistrate that P.A. be sectioned for one year in hospital [...] So because of the police he got into the hospital- otherwise he wouldn't have. Not everybody with a mental illness goes banging on a surgery door saying will you please assess me- even now they don't![25]

After receiving treatment in the psychiatric hospital, E.A. describes how her brother recovered very quickly in this care setting. When her mother first went to see P.A. in the hospital, she was worried he might blame her for his situation. However, E.A. narrates how her brother was actually able to reassure their mother saying—'it's okay here, they know what they are talking about. They understand. I'll be alright here.'[26] E.A. identifies how, 'from the time he went through those gates with the classical urns on them, he thought perhaps he could open up,' noting that 'the only person that he had ever opened up to before was me.'[27]

Talking of her experiences with the medical services in general, E.A. stated: 'So in a way we were lucky… the NHS people were brilliant, with us as a family and with P.A., and on the whole, we were really quite friendly with the CPNs. And on the whole, we have a lot to be thankful for. It isn't always the case today.'[28] Nevertheless, even with such a positive experience of mental health services, it is clear that E.A. needed more than this for reassurance and assistance for looking after her brother on a day-to-day basis. When asked what the real benefit of the National Schizophrenia Fellowship was, E.A. stated unthinkingly:

> It offered more support- I should have said that. In the beginning, the first eight years before Rethink, those first eight years or so the medical people were very good, as I told you, but we were completely on our own apart from that.[29]

This notion of being completely alone without any support is really important, and E.A. explained how this loneliness was frequently made worse by the stigma which attached itself to the diagnosis of 'schizophrenia' in the mid-1960s.

Stigma and Feelings of Loneliness

Before joining the Fellowship, E.A. often described a feeling of loneliness, which was inherently linked to the stigma which she and P.A. knew were attached to his condition. In periods of 'wellness', she argued that herself and her brother could easily conceal his diagnosis. She mentioned many of P.A.'s friends, stating 'So for 17 years these friends had no idea, and sometimes they'd say "oh P.A. is a law unto himself" or "P.A. is a bit eccentric" but that's all, nothing more. But I shouldn't have had to hide it.'[30] The halfway house of wellness and illness which could be experienced by the episodes of schizophrenia has clearly led E.A. to lead a life of silence, trying to keep her promise to her brother, whilst remaining interested and wanting to find the release of talking to others.

> Anyway P.A. said to me, "promise me, you will not ever mention anything to do with me ever being in a mental hospital to my friends." I mean they were good friends, but he didn't know how they were going to react and he wasn't going to take the chance. And do you know, even now, I'm still keeping quiet about it. I mean I do not approve of having to keep quiet about it- do you understand? I don't approve. I support Rethink, they know I do... but a promise is a promise, even when a person is no longer here. I mean if they hear obliquely about it from some other means, then I don't worry too much, but I will never say anything about it to his friends. And so really sometimes it gets a bit awkward or something and my poor old brain, you know, I think to myself sometimes I need to put my brain into gear before I open [my mouth]. He said that he didn't want me to tell anybody and I said well they may understand or know someone else who has had a breakdown, but he said, no, he doesn't want anybody to know. I said, okay, I won't tell anybody.[31]

Interestingly in the interview with E.A., it is clear that the stigma and keeping quiet were some of the hardest things about looking after her brother, harder in some respects even, than managing the illness itself. In her interview, she explains 'it was quite a big thing to cope with- who knows and who doesn't- I mean it is almost like being a hunted criminal.'[32] By comparing her life of silence surrounding her brother's illness to being a 'hunted criminal,' E.A. clearly identifies the difficulties and shame involved in her double life. Whilst E.A. saw no reason for this stigma, it is clear that she and her family had experienced it first-hand.

> You see even one or two neighbours who used to chat to mum before, when she said she met her on the street and she said oh P.A. is behaving oddly or something and when mum said "oh he's been in hospital for a mental disorder," that neighbour withdrew. And the next time that she saw mum, she walked over on the other side of the road. And this was very hurtful to mum, I mean you have enough trouble in the first place, and then that.[33]

Similarly, she mentioned that family was of little help to bear the weight of P.A.'s illness. In a characteristic defence of her relatives, E.A. added, 'I think my family were frightened [they] thought they might be expected to get involved in financial business- which they never were because I always worked and paid my way so… that we could still have a quality of life- I thought that our happiness was paramount.'[34] Nevertheless, her family's response was clearly hurtful to herself and her mother; 'But, you know, I think that mum would have been pleased if our relatives would have written occasionally just to say- "oh how's P.A.? I do hope he's getting on alright." But they seemed either embarrassed or I don't know what it was.'[35] For many years, the burden of caring responsibilities was shared between E.A. and her mother. After her mother's death however, E.A. was on her own to care for her brother for 17 years. Speaking of her feelings of isolation, E.A. argued:

> When people are very psychotic, they lose their friends, a lot of them. In fact, I will say that people not only lose their friends, but there can be distance from their relatives on both sides. I don't mean that the relatives were nasty, they were both nice families and we had happy childhoods, but mental health is too much, apparently, to come to grips with and you know, even, extended family, and so we have been more or less on our own with the medical authorities, and of course Rethink and special friends who can take it.[36]

The response of her family and the need to hide it from certain friends clearly left a gap of loneliness in E.A.'s life, unable to talk to anyone about the more troubling symptoms of her brother's illness, including his suicide attempts and periods of hospitalisation. Clearly, this left a mark of frustration on E.A. who still worries that she might break her promise to her brother to this day. These feelings of isolation, expressed by E.A. were extremely common. An article published in *Mind and Mental Health Magazine* in 1972 argued that the stigma of the illness isolated families from neighbours, communities and even their own extended families stating that the 'sheer disruptive power of schizophrenia over a family is fully intelligible only to those who have been through it.'[37]

A Plea for Action

E.A.'s narrative is interesting, but not unusual, and her family were clearly not the only family trying to look after loved ones who had been, or who were waiting to be, diagnosed with schizophrenia. In 1966, two years after P.A.'s diagnosis, it was estimated that 11,419 individuals had been discharged from hospital with a diagnosis of schizophrenia, who had not previously been in hospital before.[38] Moreover, the World Health Organization's estimate was that the risk of being diagnosed with schizophrenia was one per cent of the population as a whole.[39] In 1970, it was observed that over half of all of the patients in mental hospitals or psychiatric units on any given day are diagnosed as suffering from schizophrenia. At the end of 1970, the number of schizophrenic patients in hospitals totalled around 58,000.[40] If anything, E.A.'s experiences, certainly those which have been recounted in the interview, were more positive than other stories appear to have been. However, the themes of isolation and loneliness prevail in other narratives too.[41] On 9 May 1970, an article featured in *The Times*. It took the form of a letter, and although it was published anonymously, it was written by a man named John Pringle. Pringle was a retired university professor, and he was also the father of a young man who had been diagnosed with Schizophrenia in his early twenties. The letter was a plea for action, a call to know that there were others out there who engaged in the same daily battles: battles not only against the illness of schizophrenia, but against the authorities, against the system, against the stigma of the illness and against the isolation that the condition created. In the letter, it is clear to hear the anguish and anger of a man, alone in a fiercely difficult situation. In the letter, he explains:

> The word "schizophrenia" is flung about today with flip facility, bobbing up in films, television scripts, literary criticism, even political articles, mostly as some sort of modish synonym for indecisiveness. But no one who has seen the acute medical condition would ever want to use it except in its correct context.[42]

In his second year at Oxford University, Pringle's son had developed what was referred to as 'depression of adolescence.' Having lost his scholarship through poor attendance, he was eventually expelled from the university and sent back to live with his worried, and until that point, completely ignorant parents.

> A family suddenly faced with this situation has, in my experience, two problems, and it is hard to say which is worst. The first is how best to cope with this strange, new member of the household whose moods alternate impossibly between sullen lying on his bed in the dark to wild fits of aggression, with social manners regressed to an almost animal level.

> The second problem is how to penetrate the obfuscating fog of hospital vagueness and evasiveness to obtain intelligible guidance on the first set of problems.[43]

Pringle's letter was a heartfelt plea of a man unable to know what action to take next. In similarity to the narrative that E.A. presents, Pringle's letter identified that positive diagnosis of schizophrenia took over two years. Pringle describes this as a time where his family were unable to receive any 'practical sense out of anybody.' Practicalities were certainly an issue of constant worry and concern for Pringle, who wrote of his frustration at not being able to find any suitable answers 'on almost any specific point on which advice was desperately needed.'[44] The letter observes the frustration in the lack of communication, but predominantly lack of advice available to family members or caregivers who found themselves suddenly in an impossible situation, with a moral duty to provide care, but a lack of communication from the medical authorities, upon whom they were reliant for information and support to uphold this responsibility. Again feelings of isolation were dominant in this narrative of caregiving, and similarly to the narrative put forward by E.A., Pringle's letter suggested the segregation that he felt as more people 'gave up' on his son and his son's condition.

> Schizophrenics tend to leave behind them a trail of people who righteously or despairingly, feel they have "done as much as we can" and it should be somebody else's turn. I have quite a collection of sympathetic letters "hoping your son's condition will soon improve" while regretfully saying "no" to some specific request.[45]

By comparing the schizophrenic patient to other classes of the disabled, Pringle suggested that they and, therefore by association, the family or caregivers 'excite none of the sympathy which surrounds other classes of the disabled.'[46] In total, the letter incited more than four hundred replies from people who were touched and moved by his words, feeling themselves in similar situations. In reference to the replies that he received, Pringle stated that he 'became involved in a remarkable volume of correspondence which opened my eyes to the sense of isolation and hopelessness to which many families up and down the country [were] living.'[47] As a result of this correspondence, the idea was formulated to look into the option of setting up a 'small group or society, primarily of relatives and other non-medical people, specifically devoted to schizophrenia, with the aim of helping families to cope with the manifold problems of the condition.'[48] The letters clearly echoed the emotions felt by E.A. and Pringle.[49]

Whilst some of the letters acknowledged that parents and relatives had approached existing mental health charities such as the N.A.M.H for help, often authors felt alone and wanted something practical to be achieved. As early as 20 July 1970, Pringle wrote to Christopher Mayhew, N.A.M.H's Chair and serving Labour MP at the House of Commons to ask for his thoughts and advice about the proposed pressure group. Setting out his desires and explanation for the necessity of such a group, Pringle observed, 'I do not believe that the kind of group that I have in mind would in any way duplicate the work which the N.A.M.H is already doing, still less cut across it.'[50] In a competitive world of the charitable sector, gaining approval from one of the biggest 'rival' associations was an important first step. This also suggests that the merger of the original charities who amalgamated to form the N.A.M.H had failed in its ability to remain personal.[51] In his private collection, Pringle meticulously kept the notes of the families who had originally contacted him, with any information that these individuals had supplied about their attempts to elicit help from local authorities or charitable bodies. Interestingly, noted under one of these families is the line, 'asked N.A.M.H if they would arrange a meeting for relatives, but they would not.'[52] On the 22 July 1970, Pringle wrote to another M.P. and Chairman of the Association of Psychiatric Work (APSW), Mary Lane, again asking for advice, this time referring to his endeavours at trying to get a 'self-help group started.'[53] Clearly, the desire to start a self-help group came from the feelings of the lack of help available elsewhere, even from existing mental health charitable bodies.

Feelings of Support

One of the many people who saw the letter in *The Times* and felt strongly enough to answer was E.A. Her brother, P.A., was living at home at the time, but had been diagnosed for many years. In answer to the question, 'how did you get involved in Rethink?' E.A. answered:

> Well, it was about 8 years after P.A. had to go into hospital... I saw a letter, in *The Times*, and it was from a Mr Pringle. It was outlining the crises going on in mental health and his experiences [...] When I saw this letter,

> it so resonated with often how we were feeling and how it could be also with other people that I wrote to the PO Box number which they gave us. Mr and Mrs Pringle invited me to go over there one evening, which I did and they were very nice. And we had a discussion about it and we decided that although it was difficult to get help from the authorities, it was side-lined, in our opinion, we would make an effort ourselves to form a group- a pressure group. And at first we called it the Schizophrenia Action Committee.[54]

Explaining the growth of the support group in its early stages, E.A. continued:

> By the second meeting we decided that... it would not in fact be done in five minutes so we changed the name to the [National] Schizophrenia Fellowship, but we still had the same aims. So that is what we did- I still have my first membership card- and from that meeting other things followed and the word got around and we managed to do meetings in either one of the houses. There were quite a few people who had relatives affected like us, and we grew and grew.[55]

The first exploratory meeting was held on 25 July 1970 at the Wellcome Building on Euston Road.[56] Pringle chaired the meeting, and it was decided that steps should be taken, primarily through advertising, to find out how many 'relatives of schizophrenics and others interested would be prepared to join a Schizophrenia Society, if formed.'[57] Interestingly, whilst the meeting unanimously decided that it wanted its membership to be 'as far reaching as possible,' from the very beginning, this was a society for relatives, rather than specifically for those suffering from schizophrenia themselves.[58] It was stated that the 'prime objectives of a schizophrenia society would be to bring help and support to relatives of schizophrenics and to improve public provision, and to enhance knowledge.'[59] Indeed, one of their main original aims, in addition to lobbying the government for change, was to 'run a counselling service for relatives.'[60] It was even questioned in the first meeting whether membership of the society should be solely limited to close relatives and parents of schizophrenics. This suggestion was not taken up; it was decided instead in favour of allowing mental health specialists and others with a specialist interest to partake in membership.[61] Nevertheless, despite the inclusion of specialists, it is clear that relatives were the primary membership and the real reason for the establishment of the society.

The idea that the Fellowship was able to bring relatives and caregivers together was amongst its key success. Together, it was felt that they were able to look after each other and beat the stigma of schizophrenia. This was amongst the main aim of the society when it was first established. It was felt that 'since the feelings of loneliness by those coping with schizophrenia may sometimes be helped by meeting and talking to others who are, or who have been, in the same case, it might be possible to arrange local or area meetings.'[62] By October 1975, these local meetings were in successful operation. It was noted that these group meetings were spaces 'in which problems could be discussed, and members provided with advice, support and mutual companionship.'[63] In this way, during these meetings, the National Schizophrenia Fellowship allowed E.A. to open up and be able to talk to people in a safe and non-judgemental environment. Here, she was able to talk about her difficulties and about her brother, safe in the knowledge that here, her promise could remain unbroken.

> When these meetings started up, you felt quite cheered up, you felt positive; it was something. You felt like you were doing something and that we would get there somehow and it was so nice to be able to open up to people instead of pussy-footing around all the time- I had got fed up with it and that was a very strong development eight years after P.A. was diagnosed in his condition. At last I had met other people in the same position and we didn't judge each other or anything so that is a very strong thing that Rethink do- getting people together.[64]

On 6 October 1975, the NSF could claim that it had over 1000 members, reaching nearly 1500 individuals.[65] It was boasted that the Fellowship had members across the UK, in Northern Ireland and the Irish Republic. Talks were even being held to try to set up similar fellowships in New Zealand, Japan and South Africa.[66] By the Annual General Meeting of February 1976, there were sixty local NSF groups established in local districts.[67] The chairman stated his pride that already these groups' 'views and needs were been listened to and even sought after by staffs of the Health and Social Services. Individual members had found that they could offer each other help, advice and mutual companionship which they had often been without for many years.'[68] One member was quoted as having stated 'how marvellous' the NSF was, claiming 'I want to jump on my roof-top and shout out that I have schizophrenia in my family after twenty years of isolation.'[69] However, it was clear that this was just the beginning and they already had plans to grow their number of sixty support groups. Future plans were not only to increase the number, but also to increase the scope of the work of these local groups. The Annual Report identified that 'the local groups were looking towards an intensification of self-help, befriending, sitting in, arranging holidays and so on…'[70] E.A. explains;

> From then, we had a donation from somebody, I don't know if I should mention their name but they were very well respected in the science world and the banking world and they gave us about £3000 to set up an official [head-quarters] - she herself was affected by a relative and that money helped us to set up an office in Surbiton at the time. So little by little it has grown. We set up support groups in various areas and then we tried to make it nationwide. And they seem to me to have done a good job.[71]

Members received a variety of benefits for their £2.50 subscription money. They were entitled to receive a regular newsletter, pamphlets and leaflets setting out practical guidance for looking after relatives with the disease. Families were also entitled to membership at a local group meeting. The Member's Pamphlet explained that members would benefit from the 'sense of belonging to a national society run by relatives *for* relatives, whose sole purpose is to secure a better life for people with schizophrenia and their families.'[72] In this way, the Fellowship was ardently set up as an organisation not solely for the benefit of the schizophrenic, but as a release valve and coping mechanism for the healthy-minded relative being pushed into an unhealthy life of anxiety and isolation by the illness.

Better Together

Despite being positive of her own experiences of the medical professionals, E.A. was exceptionally critical about any attempt to undercut funding and reduce services available for mental health work. Her membership of the National Schizophrenia Fellowship allowed her access to Service Review Meetings, and she was critical here of the mindset of reducing services to cut costs in the mental health budget.[73]

> I was asked to go along, not because I was a medical person, but because a social services for Hammersmith Mental Health Occupation Therapist asked me to go along, as her sidekick I suppose you might call it, because

> she said that I might be able to say things that she as an employee of the council might not be able to say. And I remember at one time I really was incensed because they said that various inspectors had been going around and they had seen nurses playing table tennis with a patient and they were regarding it as messing about- really(!)- They were not regarding this as therapy! So they were obviously thinking that nurses themselves were not on duty- they had not got the mind-set and I was worried. This was before the mental hospitals had closed, just as they were coming up for closure and I remember saying- to someone-they were trying to work out how they could have the minimum in the community- the minimum number of CPNs and when I questioned it they said "it's all very well, but there isn't the money in the NHS and we have got to keep in our budget and we just can't afford to have CPNs playing noughts and crosses ... we just cannot afford it." And I said to them... "if you want successful community care for people who are mentally ill, you cannot afford not to... They must be there!" There was a long silence. Nobody said anymore. The meeting went on. I was never asked again to the service review but the Occupational Therapist said to me, "I am so glad that you said that- I couldn't have said that... but you're independent."[74]

In other respects, the National Schizophrenia Fellowship was an important body which lobbied the government to change the system. The Annual Reports document work carried out and early reports set the tone for encouraging change. The early publication, *The Problem Before Us*, set out the Fellowship's claim for the deficiencies in caring for those with schizophrenia. The document listed a range of issues that needed addressing, such as inadequate spending on research, negative public attitudes and stigma towards the illness, ignorance of mental illness amongst general practitioners and a basic unfamiliarity with committal procedures amongst general practitioners, amongst many.[75] In turn, the ideas behind this work came from the problems identified in Pringle's original letter, which was so powerful in terms of finding publicity in *The Times*. The early pressure group focused on trying to rectify some of the issues put forward in Pringle's original letter, which highlighted the need for a 'unified national policy' when it came to trying to deal with the problem of schizophrenia. Much time and effort was put into the charity's efforts to arrange 'small residential settlements' where the schizophrenic's basic needs could be provided for. In turn, the benefits being fought for would have had a huge impact on the families and caregivers of individuals with schizophrenia. These ideas culminated in a report of recommendations submitted to the Secretary of State, Barbara Castle, on the 'Social Provision for Sufferers from Chronic Schizophrenia.'[76]

By the late 1970s, a host of different pamphlets and publications had been made available by the NSF. These were originally designed for members only; however, it soon became apparent that they could attract a 'good deal of publicity.' The brochure entitled *Schizophrenia* had been handed to the national press, and this had led to a huge demand from general practitioners and social workers.[77] Further interviews in the national press led to publicity on the television, and information provided by the Fellowship was screened as part of a 'Horizon' documentary on BBC2 in March 1974. All of this publicity meant that the Fellowship was able to grow, both in terms of a pressure group, but also in their influence nationally as well as in individual families.

These pamphlets were designed very specifically to meet a perceived gap in the market for knowledge. Early in his endeavours to set up the Fellowship, Pringle wrote: 'The bewilderment and loneliness of relatives trying to make sense of the appalling thing that hits them is being helped very little, if at all. The BMA [British Medical Association] and the N.A.M.H. have leaflets for relatives of a primarily soothing and not very adequate kind. The society are starting hopes to do better than this.'[78] Talking about the impact that Rethink has on her modern day life, E.A. identifies that the explanation of medical information is now one of the things she values the most.

> What I value about in their journal, *Your Voice*, is all the information about new medications coming on, because they do help. So I very much enjoy reading about scientific developments and they are very good at that- fact-sheets- and things like that... that is one of the things that I still value and think how they can help two of my local friends when I read these fact-sheets. So that has a high priority with me.[79]

Whilst the pressure that the NSF was able to put on the government was not insubstantial in the late 1970s and early 1980s, this work was intensified during this period by a collection of other mental health charitable groups. The rebranded N.A.M.H., which had changed its name to MIND following a successful campaign in 1972, still had a dominant position in lobbying the government for change. It is clear from the quote above, however, that the NSF played a special role in thinking specifically about schizophrenia. The factsheets and pamphlets that they produced may have had a valuable role in increasing publicity and certainly found interest in the media at the time. However, again, it is clear that this information was the most valued by the society's membership. The fact that Pringle wanted the leaflets to be more 'adequate' for relatives and caregivers than those available by the BMA and the N.A.M.H. is very telling.

Conclusions

It is clear that to begin with, the NSF was established to respond to the loneliness, isolation and stigma felt by relatives and caregivers of those suffering from schizophrenia in the 1970s in Britain. E.A.'s story, Pringle's letter and the correspondence that he received, published in *Living with Schizophrenia: By the Relatives* in 1974, all show a remarkably similar story of individuals doing their best but suffering in relative isolation. Some people felt abandoned by family, some by friends and others by the NHS and medical staff themselves. The NSF was designed to bring these relatives and caregivers together and provide them with a voice. The Fellowship provided literature and pamphlets, explaining the illness, lobbied the government to provide change and worked with the media to try to dispel the myths and stigma surrounding schizophrenia. However, despite this work, the Fellowship itself remained one of the most important things, giving families and caregivers a voice and offering the comforting familiarity of friends who have had similar experiences. Advice was both scientific—in terms of the factsheets—but also based on human experience.

This supportive message of self-help was interconnected with every ambition of the Fellowship, including its very name. The aims of the Fellowship were cyclical; improving the life of the family member and caregiver and offering them information, advice and support would improve the life of the schizophrenic person and thereby improve the lives of their caregivers. To finish with the eloquent words of E.A. 'So whatever happens, Rethink is there and I feel that they will plug the gap. I will never forget the first time that I walked away from that first meeting- the first big meeting with lots of people there- and I thought more sort of hopeful and more normal, instead of sort of cut off from people and so that.... can all help make a difference.'[80] E.A.'s words are suggestive; it would appear that becoming a member of the NSF could help to support relatives struggling with stigma and act as a barrier to this stigma, by providing help, mutual friendship and strategies of coping for the 'healthy mind' of the non-schizophrenic caregiver.

Acknowledgements I would like to thank Mark Winstanley (Chief Executive of Rethink Mental Illness) and the people at Rethink for allowing me to access the archives and providing funding to do so. My biggest thanks go to E.A., my interviewee, for allowing me to publish this material, and being so welcoming. Your zest and enthusiasm for life is infectious.

Notes

1. NSF Archive: Schizophrenia Action Committee, 'Schizophrenia: Could You Help?' (1970).
2. Ibid.
3. Ibid. Emphasis original.
4. Brea Perry, *50 Years After Deinstitutionalisation: Mental Illness in Contemporary Societies* (London: Emerald Group Publishing Ltd, 2016); Helen Killaspy, "From the Asylum to Community Care: Learning from Experience," *British Medical Bulletin* 79, no. 1 (June 2006): 245–258; John Welshman, "Rhetoric and Reality: Community Care in England and Wales, 1948–74," in *Outside the Walls of the Asylum: The History of Care in the Community 1750–2000*, eds. Peter Bartlett and David Wright (London and New Brunswick: The Athlone Press, 1999); Peter Barham, *Closing the Asylum: The Mental Patient in Modern Society* (London: Penguin Books, 1992).
5. Dylan Tomlinson, "What Happened to the Patients?" in *Utopia, Community Care and the Retreat from the Asylums* (Milton Keynes and Philadelphia: Open University Press, 1991), 135–155.
6. Alex Mold, *Making the Patient Consumer: Patient Organisations and Health Consumerism in Britain* (Manchester: Manchester University Press, 2015), 18.
7. Ali Haggett, "Preventing Male Mental Illness in Post-war Britain," in *Preventing Mental Illness: Past, Present and Future*, eds. Despo Kritsotaki, Vicky Long, and Matthew Smith (Basingstoke: Palgrave Macmillan, 2019), 261.
8. John K. Walton, "Casting Out and Bringing Back in Victorian England, Pauper Lunatics, 1840–70," in *The Anatomy of Madness: Essays in the History of Psychiatry*, eds. W. F. Bynum, R. Porter, and M. Shepherd (London: Tavistock, 1985), 132–146.
9. David Wright, "Getting Out of the Asylum: Understanding the Confinement of the Insane in the Nineteenth Century," *Social History*

of Medicine 10, no. 1 (April 1997): 137–155; David Wright, *Mental Disability in Victorian England: The Earlswood Asylum, 1847–1901* (Oxford: Oxford University Press, 2001); Louise Wannell, "Patient's Relatives and Psychiatric Doctors: Letter Writing in the York Retreat, 1875–1910," *Social History of Medicine* 20, no. 2 (August 2007): 297–313, 297.

10. Nicole Baur, "Family Influence and Psychiatric Care: Physical Treatments in Devon Mental Hospitals c. 1920 to the 1970s," *Endeavour* 37, no. 3 (July 2013): 172–183, 177.
11. Anon, "A Case of Schizophrenia by a Correspondent," *The Times*, 9 May 1970.
12. John Pringle, "Living with Schizophrenia," *Mind and Mental Health Magazine* (Spring 1972): 15.
13. Nick Crossley, "Transforming the Mental Health Field: the Early History of the National Health Association of Mental Health," *Sociology of Health and Illness* 20, no. 4 (December 2001): 458–488.
14. Vicky Long, *Destigmatising Mental Illness? Professional Politics and Public Education in Britain, 1870–1970* (Manchester: Manchester University Press, 2014), 162.
15. NSF Archive, Personal Papers, 29 July 1970.
16. Ibid.
17. Nick Crossley, *Contesting Psychiatry: Social Movements in Mental Health* (London and New York: Routledge, 2006).
18. Barham, *Closing the Asylum*, 144.
19. For a discussion of stigma linked to mental illness, see: Long, *Destigmatising Mental Illness?*
20. A.B. Interview with E.A. recorded 11.04.2018. (Timing: 00.23:13–00:23:24).
21. E.A. accepted the use of the terms E.A. referring to herself and P.A. referring to her brother as acceptable for this publication.
22. Interview with E.A. (00:45:30).
23. Interview with E.A. (00:44:09–00:44.45).
24. Interview with E.A. (00:49:14–00:49:24).
25. Interview with E.A. (00:51:10–00.53.20).
26. Interview with E.A. (00:56:20–00:56:30).
27. Interview with E.A. (00:56:40–00:57:11).
28. Interview with E.A. (01:03:37–01:04:47).
29. Interview with E.A. (01:19:26–01:20:03).
30. Interview with E.A. (00:22:32–00:22:54).
31. Interview with E.A. (00:15:16–00:17:33).
32. Interview with E.A. (00:24:28–00:24:40).
33. Interview with E.A. (01:20:04–01:20:58).

34. Interview with E.A. (00:08:55–00:09:41).
35. Interview with E.A. (00:24:09–00:24:27).
36. Interview with E.A. (00:00:27–00:01:28).
37. John Pringle, "Living with Schizophrenia," *Mind and Mental Health Magazine* (Spring 1972), 15–20.
38. NSF Archive, *The Problem Before Us*. No date.
39. Ibid.
40. NSF Archive, Personal Correspondence, J. K. Wing to John Pringle, 3 October 1972.
41. See J. Wing and Clare Creer, *Schizophrenia at Home* (1974); Anon, *Living with Schizophrenia—By the Relatives* (1974).
42. Anon, "A Case of Schizophrenia by a Correspondent," *The Times*, 9 May 1970.
43. Ibid.
44. Ibid.
45. Ibid.
46. Ibid.
47. NSF Archive, Correspondence—John Pringle to Rt Hon. Christopher Mayhew M.P., 20 July 1970.
48. Ibid.
49. Anon, *Living with Schizophrenia*.
50. NSF Archive, Correspondence—John Pringle to Rt Hon. Christopher Mayhew M.P., 20 July 1970.
51. Long, *Destigmatising Mental Illness*, 163.
52. NSF Archive, Personal Papers, 29 July 1970.
53. NSF Archive, Correspondence—John Pringle to Rt Hon. Mrs. Lane M.P., 22 July 1970.
54. Interview with E.A. (01:10:06–01:12:39).
55. Interview with E.A. (01:12:33–01:13:49).
56. NSF Archives: Memorandum and Articles of Association of the National Schizophrenia Fellowship (September 1975).
57. Ibid.
58. Ibid.
59. NSF Archive, *The Problem Before Us*.
60. Ibid.
61. Ibid.
62. Ibid.
63. NSF Archive, General Papers, 6 October 1975.
64. Interview with E.A. (01:21:36–01:22:42).
65. Membership could include a 'family membership,' whereby one subscription would allow both a husband and wife to access resources.
66. NSF Archive, General Papers, 6 October 1975.

67. NSF Archive, Minutes of the Annual General Meeting (February 1976).
68. Ibid.
69. NSF Archive, General Papers, 6 October 1975.
70. NSF Archive, Minutes of the Annual General Meeting (February 1976).
71. Interview with E.A. (01:14:37–01:15:52).
72. NSF Archive, National Schizophrenia Fellowship, *Member's Pamphlet*, 1974. Emphasis original.
73. Interview with E.A. (00:57:30).
74. Interview with E.A. (00:58:00–01:01:49).
75. NSF Archive, *The Problem Before Us*. No date.
76. NSF Archive, *'Social Provision for Sufferers from Chronic Schizophrenia.' Recommendations, June 1974.*
77. NSF Archive, *Schizophrenia*. No date.
78. NSF Archive, Personal Correspondence to John Day, 10 May 1971.
79. Interview with E.A. (01:17:50–01:18:08).
80. Interview with E.A. (01:22:54–01:23:56).

CHAPTER 10

'(Un)healthy Minds' and Visual and Tactile Arts, c.1900–1950

Imogen Wiltshire

Introduction

During the first half of the twentieth century, there were vast changes in psychological models of the mind, new psychotherapies and physiological forms of treatment, advances in medical imaging and diagnostic technologies that probed the inner body, and a host of new allied health professions. The visual arts, including painting, drawing, craft, prints, sculpture, architecture, graphic design and photography, in Western Europe and the USA were intermeshed with methods of healing, and the concepts of the body and mind on which they were predicated, in manifold ways. Modernist architects and designers were commissioned to produce sanatoria and psychiatric institutions in line with shifting ideas about therapeutic environments. Interwar preoccupations with physical fitness and mental hygiene, which posited the holistic ideal of a healthy mind in a healthy body, were portrayed in and cultivated by visual representations of athletic bodies and sport. Art was increasingly conceptualised in the late nineteenth and early twentieth centuries as expressing

I. Wiltshire (✉)
University of Leicester, Leicester, UK
e-mail: iw61@leicester.ac.uk

S. J. Taylor and A. Brumby (eds.), *Healthy Minds in the Twentieth Century*, Mental Health in Historical Perspective,
https://doi.org/10.1007/978-3-030-27275-3_10

subjective experiences, based on growing notions of psychological interiority and the self held within. There was a developing interest in exploring the psychologically ameliorative effects of viewing art: laboratories tested the psychophysical responses elicited in participants by colour and form, while there was a growing articulation of the escapist function of visual cultural forms, especially during and after the First World War. Meanwhile visual and tactile art-making practices were instrumentalised as a means of therapy in a range of healthcare contexts in art, medical, pedagogic and psychiatric institutions in the early to mid-twentieth century.

In the context of this volume's objective to probe the plurality of domains in which mental-health care operated, this chapter explores the function of art in shaping the treatments and cultural perceptions of mental illness both within and outside psychiatric institutions conventionally associated with defining and maintaining mental health at this time. Art was understood to contribute to sustaining psychological health and to constitute a form of healing in a multitude of ways but was also an arena in which professional artists critically engaged with the practices and concepts of psychotherapeutic regimes. Indeed, existing art historical accounts that examine modern art's intersection with mental health have primarily focused on how psychoanalysis and psychiatry in particular provided a means of inspiration and subversion for canonical modern artists. In *fin-de-siècle* Vienna, where modernist art practices, mental illness and psychiatric treatments overlapped in distinctive ways, as art historian Gemma Blackshaw has shown, artist Egon Schiele, for example, was informed by pathological anatomy approaches to psychiatry, appropriating diseased bodies in his work as an avant-garde strategy.[1] Certainly, while the focus of this book is the multitude of ways in which mental health was assessed, created and maintained, some modern artists actively resisted the rationality associated with the 'healthy mind'. As is well documented in art history, a core objective of Surrealism, initiated in Paris in 1924, was to evince the irrationality and taboo of the repressed unconscious. Some Surrealists rejected psychiatry, celebrated nineteenth-century conceptions of hysteria and developed representational methods designed to invoke the subversive aspects of the psyche, informed by psychoanalysis.[2] It is precisely art's capacity to examine, transgress and critique which means that artists were not only informed by approaches to mental health and the perceived experiences of illness but also challenged and even exploited them. Examining mental health through the lens of art brings to the fore issues of power and agency centred especially on who delineates what constitutes the contingent concept of a 'healthy mind', which voices are emphasised in historical narratives and how objects pertaining to treatment, including works made therapeutically, are handled by therapists and historians.

This chapter aims to offer a broad survey that both provides new research on therapeutic uses of art and synthesises for the first time wide-ranging forms of existing literature on modern art and psychological functions in order to map multifarious and complex intersections between art practices, mental illness and mental health. The investigation concentrates, with a transnational lens, on three key thematic areas: first, how artwork by professional artists was understood to induce beneficial psychological effects in viewers; second, the celebration and appropriation by modern artists of mental illness to avant-garde ends; finally, the multifaceted ways in which art-making practices were used in the fields of occupational therapy and, later in the same century, art therapy. This chapter consequently takes a comparatively broad view of art: my concern is not only with paintings and drawings by modern artists, but also with experiential and ephemeral art and craft practices in mental-health care contexts. The ideas, practices and applications of art that take place outside art institutions generally feature less in art historical enquiry, and extending the boundaries accordingly beyond professional artists, museums and exhibitions allows both a broader and more nuanced interrogation of this subject.

One of the most pervasive fascinations on the topic of modern art and mental illness is the trope of the psychologically tormented artist, exemplified by the prevalent mythologising in scholarship and in popular culture of Vincent van Gogh's life and artwork in terms of self-mutilation and suicide.[3] The culturally constructed myth of the mad and suffering artist whose anguish is reflected in his work (I use the pronoun deliberately), a narrative critiqued by feminist art historians in particular, derives from early nineteenth-century Romantic notions of the artist as a tortured genius who operates outside of society.[4] It is neither the concern of this chapter to examine the relationships between creativity and madness nor to analyse canonical modern art psychobiographically based on evidence or speculation about an artist's mental state. Rather, it looks to elucidate historical relationships between art and mental-health care, one configuration of which includes how modern artists and art critics consciously and deliberately engaged with and drew on psychotherapies.

Viewing Art, Psychological Health and the Restorative Function of Colour and Form

The late nineteenth and early twentieth centuries saw an unprecedented interest in the psychologically stimulating and restorative effects that the visual arts could have on viewers. Pre-Freudian psychological research in France in the mid- to late nineteenth century posited the mind as a dynamic mental chamber susceptible to visual stimulation which informed the production and reception of art, architecture and design. *Fin-de-siècle* art nouveau, characterised often by curvilinear forms, was conceptualised in light of this *psychologie nouvelle* as inciting psychological experiences through visual means.[5] Concurrently, some categories of fine art by professional artists were understood to have a mentally restorative function, specifically in some cases as an antidote to the modern condition of neurasthenia, defined as nervous exhaustion that resulted from urban existence. In 1908, modern artist Henri Matisse imagined his landscape paintings as having a mentally calming effect on the viewer:

> What I dream of is an art of balance, of purity and serenity, devoid of troubling or depressing subject matter, an art which could be for every mental worker, for the businessman as well as the man of letters, for example, a soothing, calming influence on the mind, something like a good armchair which provides relaxation from physical fatigue.[6]

Compared to the later explicitly provocative forms of early twentieth-century modern art, such as the politically driven facets of Dada, launched in Zürich in 1916 and foregrounding chaos and fragmentation to articulate the upheaval and destruction of the First World War, Matisse proposed a form of art that was psychologically comforting, especially through its subject matter. Two of his most well-known artworks from this time, *The Joy of Life* (1905–06) and *Blue Nude* (*Souvenir of Biskra*) (1907), represented an imagined ideal Arcadia of a harmonious landscape with reclining and frolicking female nudes (a subject far from unusual in art), deliberately evading signs of modernity. The envisaged beneficiary of Matisse's art was, as art historian Joyce Henri Robinson notes, the bourgeois man whose nerves have been overstimulated by the modern city and mental work.[7] The delineation of neurasthenia was gendered: men could suffer from mental fatigue whereas women, considered to be more susceptible to overstimulation in the first place, were advised to avoid the city and remain in the domestic interior to protect their nervous systems.[8] The genre of pastoral landscape painting was considered an ideal means in bourgeois thought to calm the fatigued man whose nerves had been agitated, exemplified further by the artwork of artist Pierre Puvis de Chavannes such as *Pleasant Land* (1882) (Fig. 10.1). A less formally innovative artist than Matisse, Puvis' comparatively conservative landscapes, which also depicted female nudes in an imagined Arcadia, were similarly attributed contemporarily, as Robinson shows, with a mentally restorative function: a catalogue essay for a solo exhibition in 1887 declared that, on viewing the artwork, 'you are in peace and calm; what a sensation of well-being!'.[9] This conceptualisation of painting as a vehicle for psychological tranquillity against the effects of modernity, with which Matisse aligned himself, placed emphasis on the benign psychological effects of art not in a therapeutic or clinical context but as a means of maintaining the everyday mental health of middle-class art audiences. This constitutes a specific historical instance of how viewing art was understood to play a role in mental well-being, an idea that became increasingly prevalent throughout the twentieth century.

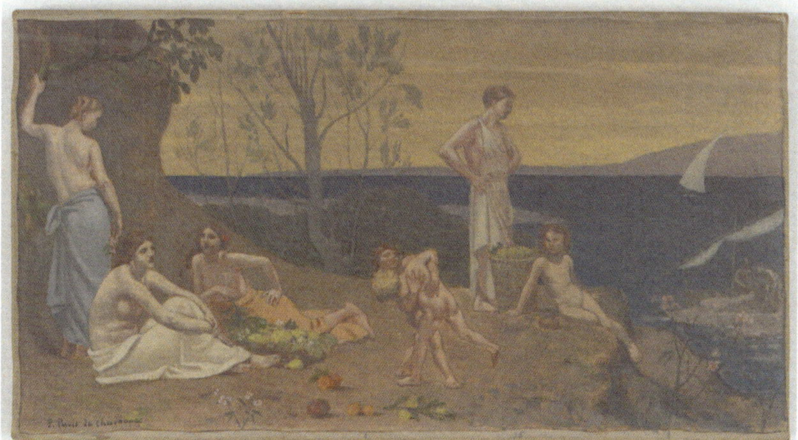

Fig. 10.1 *Pleasant Land*, 1882, Pierre Puvis de Chavannes (1824–1898). Oil on canvas, 25.7 × 47.6 cm. Photo Credit: Yale University Art Gallery. Public domain

Similarly, in Britain during the First World War, conservative pastoral landscapes in particular were conceived as a means of psychological restoration. As James Fox demonstrates, discussions of the idyllic 'peace pictures' of landscape paintings by artists including Benjamin Williams Leader, George Clausen and Tom Mostyn were inflected with concerns pertaining to mental well-being, as 'antidotes' to war that could 'purge', 'cleanse', 'heal' and 'soothe' audiences.[10] Although it is difficult to ascertain that viewers did respond to the artworks in this way, this language reveals nonetheless how conceptualisations of art and art criticism discourses were marked increasingly by an interest in psychological health.

There was a fascination in the early 1900s in the effects elicited not only by a painting's subject matter but also by its intrinsic formal properties. The psychophysiological effects that abstract qualities of colour, line and shape could have on viewers was the subject of research centred in Germany in particular. Experimental laboratories, informed by nineteenth-century theories of perception, tested the neuromuscular response of individuals to the visual stimuli of form and colour.[11] Formal properties were isolated for their potential to have an immediate and unmediated emotional effect on a person. In this context, 'simple lines and colours' came to be perceived as having 'therapeutic powers'.[12] The premise that colour especially could have a beneficial impact on human bodily functions had a precedent in nineteenth-century chromotherapy (or light therapy) in which visible, coloured light was projected onto individuals. As Tanya Sheehan has shown, a pioneer of chromotherapy was Augustus Pleasonton who developed blue-light therapy in Philadelphia during the 1870s.[13] Pleasonton posited that blue light, achieved by filtering light through panes of blue glass, had a rejuvenating power when absorbed by the cells of the body. He prescribed sunbathing under blue glass for a range of ailments including 'spinal meningitis', 'nervous debility' and 'rheumatic affections of all kinds'.[14] Working under Jean-Martin Charcot at the Salpêtrière Hospital in Paris in the late 1800s, where hysteria was intensively delineated and studied in relation to women, psychologist Charles Féré also developed a form of light therapy, glazing asylum cells with blue or violet glass in order to produce calming and curative effects.[15] While chromotherapy concerned the impact of coloured light being sensed directly by the surface of the skin, the work of Howard Kemp Prosser in medical institutions in Britain with First World War casualties centred on the therapeutic potential of inhabiting spaces decorated by particular colours. Emphasising that surroundings were integral to recovery, Prosser argued that colour itself was 'beneficial to men whose nerves have become unstrung'.[16] In line with his convictions, he organised the McCaul Ward at St John's Hospital in London and a section of the Maudsley Neurological Clearing Hospital according to his constructed colour schemes. As reported in *The British Journal of Nursing*, the wards at Maudsley had 'soft firmament blue' ceilings, 'apple-blossom pink' walls with 'anemone mauve curtains, introducing the note of concentration' and 'Spring-green quilts, the bedsteads being painted the same colour'.[17] Contemporary testimonies to the apparent efficacy of Prosser's 'colour medicine', to be approached by historians with caution, included that 'a patient with neurasthenia was cured of headaches by living in the purple room, that a man with hysteria recovered in the yellow room, and that crime was noticeably less in Prosser's coloured wards than any others'.[18]

The perceived psychophysiological effects of painting's formal properties became central to strands of modern art and aesthetic theory, most notably in the work of artist Wassily Kandinsky, widely considered a pioneer of abstract art. Kandinsky noted in his influential treatise, *On the Spiritual in Art* (*Über das Geistige in der Kunst*) (1912), that: 'anyone who has heard of colour therapy knows that coloured light can have a particular effect upon the entire body'.[19] He described how the examination of colour for 'different nervous disorders' had revealed that red light has 'enlivening and stimulating effect upon the heart' whereas blue could 'lead to temporary paralysis'. Extending similar ideas to modern art, he underscored the potential of pure colour to elicit sensory responses in the viewer. Informed by contemporary physiological psychology research, Kandinsky considered the experience of art to begin corporeally: painting first stimulated a physical vibration in the viewer's body that in turn induced a deeper spiritual vibration in the soul.[20] This response was contingent, he argued, on two factors: that the artist uses colour and form as pure composition, and, secondly, that viewers cease looking for narrative in artworks.[21] This was the context in which Kandinsky developed abstraction that extracted painting's intrinsic formal properties rather than represented recognisable figurative subject matter. His semi-abstract painting *Cossacks* (1910–11) (Fig. 10.2), for example, contains some identifiable elements, including sharp mountain forms, three cavalrymen in the right foreground, a rainbow and birds, but the compositional elements are comprised of simplified colours and shapes, and the overall perspective is flattened. Kandinsky's ideas are best

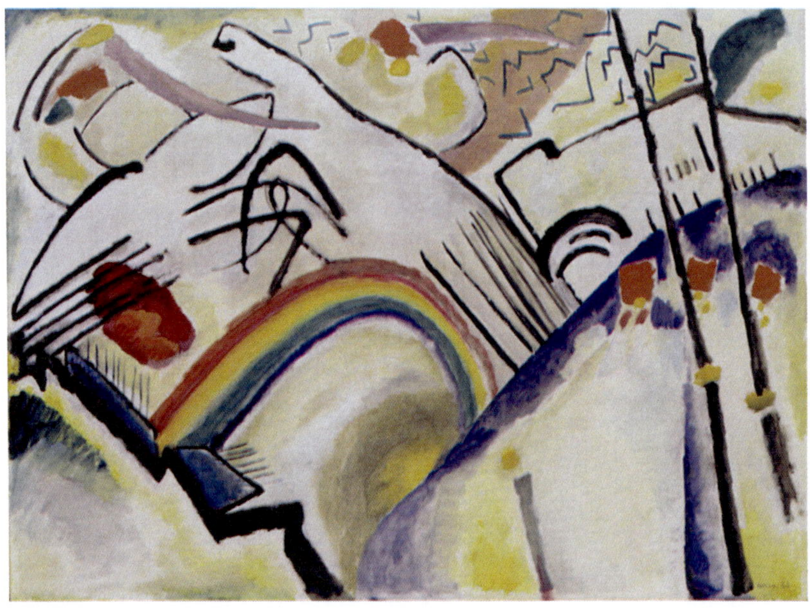

Fig. 10.2 *Cossacks*, 1910–11, Wassily Kandinsky (1866–1944). Oil on canvas, 94.6 × 130.2 cm. Presented by Mrs Hazel McKinley 1938. Photo Credit: ©Tate, London 2019.

placed within a history of modernist avant-garde interrogation of the properties and psychological effects of art, as opposed to its therapeutic application, but reveal nonetheless cross-field intersections of thought centred on art's imagined effects on viewers.

While Kandinsky's work constituted a modernist exploration that extended the boundaries of art by isolating and foregrounding its formal properties, aesthetic theories later in the twentieth century assumed and sought to explain the enduring psychological appeal of form in art. The function of creative processes and nature of aesthetic experience were central concerns in psychoanalysis-based art theory in mid-twentieth-century Britain, many aspects of which were dominated by Melanie Klein's object-relations theory. Art critic Adrian Stokes theorised the attraction of form in painting psychoanalytically using Klein's theoretical base of the two phases that constituted the formation of the ego: the paranoid-schizoid position, dominated by 'part objects', and the subsequent depressive position characterised by ego integration and a desire for reparation. Attempting to account for the appeal of art galleries, Stokes argued that, irrespective of the subject matter, form in painting was a mode of repairing the inner world and was analogous to psychic integration.[22] Contending that art assisted with the drive towards psychic reparation, he asserted that visual aesthetic experience was inherently beneficial. Stokes assumed a universal pleasure and psychological satisfaction in the viewing of art, and he accounted for this abiding mental appeal theoretically using Kleinian psychoanalytic thought. Considered together, these divergent instances demonstrate the multifaceted interest in the effects of viewing art in relation to psychological health, indicating both the expanded function of art and the extended reach of mental-health care discourses at this time.

Modern Art, Madness and Appropriating Mental Illness

Concurrent to early to mid-twentieth-century explorations of the benign psychological effects of painting on viewers, there was an avant-garde resistance to the rationality connected with the notion of a 'healthy mind'. The most prominent and sustained modernist interrogation of the irrational and illogical components of the psyche was offered by Surrealism, a movement launched in Paris in 1924, the year in which André Breton published the first 'Manifesto of Surrealism'. Embracing a diverse set of artistic practices, Surrealist artists were concerned with mental investigation, rejected intellectual and political conventions and criticised capitalist and nationalist powers. Breton had become acquainted with Sigmund Freud's psychoanalytic theories of the unconscious which had been translated into French in the 1920s. Inspired by the Freudian model of the mind as comprising repressed fantasies, anxieties, urges and desires, artists including Max Ernst, Salvador Dalí, Joan Miró, André Masson and Hans Bellmer consciously sought out and probed the 'darker' and at times sinister elements of the psyche and developed representational strategies designed to evince the illogical, the taboo, the erotic and the subversive elements of the mind. Attempting to translate the unconscious into visual representation and to foreground chance encounter, Masson and Miró, for example, engaged in automatic drawing and painting whereby the hand was allowed to move freely without conscious control, notwithstanding the deliberate additions that each artist made to their work afterwards. The Surrealists' interest in dreams as a manifestation of repressed desires is exemplified by Dalí's highly contrived and carefully composed dreamscape paintings, including one of his most well-known works, *The Persistence of Memory* (1931) with his now familiar melting clocks. Ironically perhaps, given that facets of early Surrealism were concerned with rejecting forms of institutional power, Dalí was later commissioned in 1958 by Carter-Wallace, a US drug manufacturer, to create a series of paintings to advertise the first 'tranquiliser', a sedative called Miltown (Meprobamate pharmaceutically). The artist subsequently designed an image, *Crisalida* (1958), used in a brochure that visualised the transition from psychological agitation to tranquillity effected by the drug. That the rise of the pharmaceutical companies in the mid-twentieth century generated such commercial opportunities for artists attests further to the wide-ranging relationships between the visual arts and mainstream mental-health systems.

As art historians have well documented, in line with interwar Surrealism's revolutionary objectives, psychic failure was perceived and seized upon by artists and writers as a positive subversion of established norms and social confines.[23] Deployed as an avant-garde strategy, the appropriation and celebration of mental illness took a number of forms: foregrounding mental illness in texts and artworks, adopting the persona of the 'madman', valorising the 'art of the insane' and criticising the institution of psychiatry. An historical illness that captured the Surrealist imagination was nineteenth-century hysteria, a category which was in disrepute by the 1920s but was revived by the Surrealists as a transgressive mechanism. As analysed by Briony Fer, the 'fiftieth anniversary of hysteria' was commemorated in 1928 in the journal *La Révolution Surréaliste* which reproduced photographs of a woman, deemed hysterical by Charcot at the Salpêtrière, apparently in convulsion.[24] In the accompanying text, Breton and poet Louis Aragon placed emphasis on what they saw as hysteria's insightful, creative and subversive potential: 'hysteria is by no means a pathological symptom and can in every way be considered a supreme form of expression'.[25] The Surrealists also constructed, foregrounded and identified with the 'madman' as someone marginalised by society and possessing special insights. Surrealist Antonin Artaud described this figure as 'a man whom society did not want to hear and whom it wanted to prevent from uttering certain intolerable truths'.[26] Breton, who was portrayed in a straightjacket in an etching by Max Ernst in 1923, aligning poet with patient, declared in the first Surrealist manifesto: 'I could spend my whole life prying loose the secrets of the insane'.[27] The premise that a form of truth was located in insanity and that the madman functioned as a means to view society anew was central to a sonnet entitled 'Schizophrenia' by the Dadaist and expressionist Hugo Ball. He located himself in the poem as the patient, deploying, as Sander Gilman argues, the identity of the mad poet as an 'exotic' device to critique society.[28] This invocation of the madman was not exclusive to Dada and Surrealism: the Futurists, who operated in Italy before the First World War, rejected tradition and advocated the speed and machines of modernity as subjects in art, claimed in the collective 'Futurist Painting: Technical Manifesto' (1910): 'the name of "madman" with which it is attempted to gag all innovators should be looked upon as a title of honour'.[29] By emphasising the voices of the 'mad' and highlighting the peripheral position of the mentally ill in society, modern artists, to some extent, valorised the perspectives of those inside psychiatric institutions. This identification and privileging was, however, primarily a self-serving avant-garde strategy in which the suffering experienced by the mentally ill was seemingly to a large extent overlooked.

The Surrealist movement's investment in mental illness as a creative and subversive means was also constituted through celebrating, collecting and exhibiting the 'art of the insane.' This aesthetic category comprised drawings and paintings by patients in asylums who had been given art materials usually for diversional, as opposed to therapeutic, purposes; Josef Karl Rädler, for example, a patient at Mauer-Öhling psychiatric hospital near Vienna from 1905 until his death in 1917, was provided with materials to keep 'him out of trouble'.[30] The largest and most influential collection of the 'art of the insane' was assembled by art historian and psychiatrist Hans Prinzhorn who, in 1919, began to amass objects from asylums across Germany, Italy, Switzerland and Austria. Prinzhorn subsequently published his book *Bildnerei der Geisteskranken* (*Artistry of the Mentally Ill*) (1922) which categorised and analysed works in the collection.[31] Prinzhorn considered the works to occupy an ambiguous position between art and diagnostic material: 'Bildnerei' connoted 'picture-making' rather than art (Kunst) but he also argued that, once separated from the maker or their diagnosis, an object could not be understood to reflect a specific mental illness. Considered at the time of their production largely as institutional ephemera, the redefinition of this work as 'art' was the result of interwar exhibitions and collecting practices that generated a market for such objects.[32] Modernist artists including Paul Klee, Max Ernst and Alfred Kubin saw the Prinzhorn collection, read his text, collected and displayed similar objects and, in some cases, copied the paintings and drawings stylistically.[33] The 'art of the insane' was celebrated as supposedly visionary and unfettered by academic conventions, seen to constitute free, impulsive and spontaneous acts of creativity. This assessment coincided with early twentieth-century modernist re-evaluations of the non-western 'primitive' and of artwork by children as similarly possessing special insight and creative impulse. This constituted a rejection and reappraisal of nineteenth-century theories of degeneracy which had viewed the mentally ill, the 'primitive' and children as insufficiently developed and, consequently, had considered their drawings and paintings as symptomatic of deviation. One of the earliest collections of works by the 'insane' was assembled by psychiatrist and anthropologist Cesare Lombroso in the late nineteenth century who viewed the objects primarily as visual evidence of mental pathology.[34] In contrast, Prinzhorn's collection, to some extent, as Catherine de Zegher suggests, 'advocated for the aesthetic legitimacy of the works drawn by psychotic individuals who were marginalised by society'.[35] The collection placed artistic and, ultimately, economic value on the work of psychiatric patients. This appropriation nonetheless idealised the experience of mental illness, as Gilman eloquently stresses: 'Prinzhorn's patients were ill. They were not shamans speaking an unknown tongue, nor were they Romantic artists expressing through their art conscious disapproval of modern society. These patients were ill, and their artistic productions reflected the pain and anguish caused by that illness. This fact was often overlooked by earlier commentators on the art of the mentally ill as well as by those writers who used the persona of the mad as their alter ego'.[36] The perception, moreover, of the 'art of the insane' as 'expressionist', 'visionary' and 'transgressive', on which its popularity rested, was in the first place largely a fiction constructed for avant-garde ends.[37]

Interwar and mid-twentieth-century exhibitions on Surrealism juxtaposed examples of modern art with the 'art of the insane' in order to suggest positive affinities between the two.[38] In November 1937, *Surrealist Objects and Poems* (London Gallery) displayed artworks by artists including Paul Nash, Julian Trevelyan and Eileen Agar alongside what were problematically described in the catalogue as 'objects by a schizophrenic lunatic'.[39] A seminal exhibition staged at the Museum of Modern Art (MoMA, New York), *Fantastic Art, Dada and Surrealism* (1936–1937), comprising almost seven hundred objects, similarly included works simply categorised as 'psychopathic watercolours and drawings'. The inclusion in *Fantastic Art* of both 'the art of children and the insane' as 'comparative material' alongside 'works by mature and normal artists' was explicated by curator Alfred Barr in the catalogue as follows: 'children and psychopaths exist [...] in a world of their own unattainable to the rest of us [...] Surrealist artists try to achieve a comparable freedom of the creative imagination'.[40] In other words, parallels were drawn between the creative insights achieved by modern artists and the inherently visionary and liberated perception of children and the mentally ill, who were positioned as occupying a place outside the parameters of 'normal'. While this comparison was drawn to articulate the innovation of Surrealism and the exceptional creative insight of its artists, a clear opposition was concurrently set up, however, between the creative intentionality of named modern artists and the uncontrolled instinctive activity of the unnamed mentally ill. The Surrealists differed, claimed the text, 'in one fundamental way' because 'they are perfectly conscious of the difference between the world of fantasy and the world of reality, whereas children and the insane are often unable to make this distinction'.[41] This caveat indicates a fundamental problematic of the 'primitive': while avant-garde modern artists were framed as operating intentionally, those viewed as 'primitive' were conceived as simply working instinctively and were consequently denied agency, authority and intentionality as makers.

In summary, the Surrealists drew attention to the marginalisation of psychiatric patients and questioned pathological definitions of abnormality, but this embrace of 'insanity' was primarily as a source of creative inspiration and a vehicle to criticise the confines of social and political structures, predicated on a mythologising and idealising of mental illness. At the same time, however, some Surrealists also condemned the institution of psychiatry in a way that is indicative of the capacity of the arts to produce and shape cultural meanings around mental-health care. An open letter to the directors of asylums published in *La Révolution Surréaliste* criticised psychiatry as a repressive, incarcerating and restraining institution: 'the madhouse, under cover of science and justice, is comparable to a barracks, a prison, a penal colony'.[42] The Surrealists were, according to art historian David Lomas, the 'anti-psychiatry movement of their day'.[43] Although the artists romanticised mental illness, their criticisms of the psychiatric institution had aspects in common with the sustained attacks that took place in the 1960s levelled at the categorising, silencing and controlling mechanisms of psychiatry.

Art and Craft-Making Practices as Occupational Therapy

Shifting attention away from canonical modern art and art institutions, the following discussion considers the formulation of art-making practices as a means of therapy in healthcare, rehabilitation and pedagogic contexts, a comparatively under-researched area in art history.[44] The field of occupational therapy developed as an allied health profession in the early to mid-twentieth century in which patients were prescribed creative practices as therapy, such as weaving, embroidery, woodwork, leatherwork and print-making. Tactile and visual art forms were applied across medical specialities for both physiological and psychological purposes. Occupational therapists advocated, however, holistic approaches to illness and treatment and, as such, undertaking arts and crafts was often considered to have a psychological purpose even when designated physiologically. As psychiatrist Alfred Solomon put it: 'whether or not psychiatric orders are given, a physical therapy is psychotherapeutic in character'.[45] In line with this, block-print fabric painting, according to an orthopaedic account from 1938, impacted on finger flexion and on pronation and supination of the forearm but also, psychologically, left 'little room' for 'personal broodings'.[46] Creative practices were adapted for different needs: weaving in psychiatry, for example, could involve repetitious rhythmic movements using dull colours for a sedative effect, whereas interesting 'pattern' with 'various shades of red and yellow' could stimulate the participant.[47] Occupational therapy was theorised in journals from different disciplinary directions by therapists, physicians, artists, pedagogues, psychiatrists, psychoanalysts and nurses, with its effects measured in a multitude of ways, including strengthening muscles, increasing concentration and self-confidence and developing positive habit formation. Claims about the interest aroused in patients and their appetite for participation should, however, be approached with some caution. In the context of rehabilitation in the USA after the First World War, historian Ana Carden-Coyne has shown that although articles and images published by hospitals, voluntary organisations and the White House stressed harmonious relationships between supposedly compliant disabled ex-servicemen and medical staff, some veterans resented rehabilitation and refused to participate in occupational therapy.[48] While institutional material is crucial for understanding how practices were perceived to operate, often undocumented in these records are the perspectives and experiences of participants themselves, including their possible resistance.

Occupational therapy was first developed, as Virginia Quiroga explains in her survey history, within women-led reform initiatives in the USA during the 1910s when early pioneers advocated that supervised arts and crafts could be used to treat tuberculosis, arthritis and neurasthenia, as well as industrial injuries.[49] The professionalisation and institutionalisation of the field happened slightly later in Britain: Elizabeth Casson founded the first accredited training school, Dorset House, in Bristol in 1930. Prior to this, Gartnavel Royal Asylum in Glasgow was the first institution in Britain to open an occupational therapy department in 1923, offering at first 'simple woodwork, basketry, cane chair making, raffia and pine needlework, china painting, metalwork, rugmaking, embroidery and decorative colour craft work'.[50] As the asylum's occupational therapy department grew, tasks were differentiated and patients were divided into distinct classes 'according to mental condition and prescribed occupation'.[51] An advertisement for an occupational therapist at Gartnavel in the *Lancet* in 1924 asked for a 'well-educated, intelligent, refined girl'.[52] As this call suggests, the profession was considered to be one best suited to women, based on socially constructed and prescribed gender assumptions which attributed them with the qualities of obedience and self-sacrifice to support such adjunctive treatments. As historian Beth Linker notes, well into the twentieth century occupational therapists, like nurses, maintained the 'Victorian roots' of their roles, based on nineteenth-century views that women were 'the weaker yet more nurturing sex'.[53] Indeed, the profession was still considered in the 1940s to be suited to a woman who was, according to one article, ideally: 'sensitive to herself and to others, emotionally responsive [...] of few words, of good judgment, and of a comfortable disposition'.[54]

Early occupational therapy in the 1910s was based on two core premises: that healing could arise through productive occupation and that art and craft practices were intrinsically restorative. In view of how mental-health care has been shaped by a multitude of fields, it is significant that these predicates were derived from education reform principles and the Arts and Crafts movement that originated in Britain in the 1860s and 1870s. The Arts and Crafts movement was associated most prominently with designer, writer and activist William Morris and theorist and art critic John Ruskin, who both advocated a unity between labour and art, driven by concerns about the detrimental effects of capitalist industrial production. They argued that machine-made objects were impersonal and offered no pleasure to the maker or the user.

In contrast, handwork was restorative: pleasure in the process of making by hand would lead to pleasure not only in that object but also in other aspects of life. Accordingly, arts and crafts proponents promoted the revival of traditional handicrafts and hand-made decorative and applied arts, including tapestries, furniture, ornaments and furnishings. These ideas and practices were disseminated internationally by societies, guilds and workshops, including the Chicago Arts and Crafts Society in the US which was formed at social-reform settlement Hull House in 1897. Co-founded by Jane Addams and Ellen Gates Starr in 1889, Hull House was a secular community that sought to improve the social, health and economic conditions of working-class areas of Chicago. At the centre of women-led reform, Hull House was a meeting point for organisations and social projects that shaped the development of occupational therapy.[55] Handicrafts were central to the educational programmes at Hull House as a means to withstand the tyranny of the machine and to revive work as a pleasurable process. Aiming to alleviate the alienation and tensions that workers were considered to experience, the Hull House Labour Museum enabled working-class women to engage in textile work, for example. Emphasis on the benefits of hand-making individualised objects, on the importance of pleasure in work and on creativity as an essential component of wellness were subsequently central to the therapeutic application of arts and crafts.

As occupational therapy developed, its institutionalisation was contingent on an alliance with mainstream medicine, an association that was not, however, entirely frictionless. A key symbol of the field's status as a modern healthcare profession was that occupation was prescribed by physicians and psychiatrists, a process which located the arts and crafts at the junction of art and medicine, as both creative and therapeutic practice.[56] The accredited training of therapists was divided between instruction in arts and crafts and, for example, anatomy, physiology, first aid and psychology. The position and perception of arts and crafts as instruments of treatment were not, though, entirely unequivocal in the 1930s and 1940s. One tension, as Ruth Ellen Levine notes, was that while scientific reductionist approaches to treatment increasingly divided medicine into specialisms, occupational therapists maintained a holistic approach, underpinned by its Arts and Crafts and reform pedagogy origins.[57] For some therapists, the perception of craft as frivolous and superfluous undermined occupational therapy's claim to a modern scientific paradigm. One way to articulate the success of occupational therapy, especially in its infancy, had been to demonstrate a patient's mastery of a craft and the artistic quality of the work they had produced. To this end, Gartnavel hospital reported in the mid-1920s on the 'greater proficiency [...] attained' by patients and the 'aesthetic' quality of the resultant objects.[58] Foregrounding the aesthetic value of a craft object, however, risked undermining the therapeutic imperatives and medical legitimacy of the profession. In 1944, one occupational therapist described their desire to avoid being 'damned once more with the "Arty-Crafty" label'.[59] Another therapist, Mary Atwater, argued that the purpose was 'not to produce a good basket [or] rag rug [...] but a cured patient'.[60] She minimised the significance of the objects produced to emphasise the overarching therapeutic objective of recovery. Eventually, the creative paradigm of occupational therapy was replaced in the 1960s by a functional basis concerned mostly with social assessments and activities of daily living.[61] With fewer patients treated as mental hospital in-patients and shorter hospital stays, occupational therapy was refocused in the second half of the twentieth century on discharge planning, domestic independence and community events rather than on creative practices.

Art Therapy: Painting, Expression and Agency

Another field, distinct from occupational therapy, in which visual art practices were applied to create and sustain healthy minds was art therapy, a field which was developed in Britain and the USA during the 1930s and 1940s and professionalised in the 1950s and 1960s.[62] Unlike the broad remit of occupational therapy, art therapy focused on fine art: painting, drawing and, to a lesser extent, sculpture. Compared to craft practices that usually involved following defined procedures or copying established models, art therapy tended to comprise what was perceived to be a freer kind of painting, including the representation of imagined subjects. As a result, it was more closely associated with articulating an inner self. Informed in part by the Freudian wave of the 1920s and 1930s that consolidated the idea of art as an articulation of the unconscious, which was disseminated and popularised further by mainstream Surrealism as we saw above, early art therapy was based broadly on the notion of art as a means of self-expression. What was considered to constitute 'expression' was not monolithic and varied between programmes, but early art therapists operated broadly on the premise that art alleviated tensions by releasing internal psychological forces or traumatic memories or acted as a means to communicate visually something that might not be articulated in words. The main purpose of art therapy, however, was not usually to generate images that could be read diagnostically. Emphasis was directed on the psychologically healing effects of the art-making process, rather than what might be extrapolated subsequently from resultant images. This focus on the therapeutic as opposed to diagnostic potential of art differentiated art therapy from psychoanalytic approaches prevalent in the 1930s and 1940s in which works by patients were treated as case material, simplified reductively as illustrations of psychoanalytic mechanisms.[63] Concurrent psychopathological approaches similarly examined how art could manifest mental illness symptoms visually. At Maudsley Hospital during the 1930s, Erich Guttmann and Walter Maclay characterised drawings by schizophrenic patients, arguing that psychiatric disorder could be read in the individual components and composition of an image.[64] Unlike psychoanalytic and psychopathological positioning of patient-made visual material as manifestations of mental disorder, art therapy centred on the psychologically curative possibilities derived from making art.

Artist and educator Adrian Hill first coined the term 'art therapy' in Britain in 1942 to describe his work at King Edward VII Sanatorium in Midhurst. According to Hill's own account, he offered initially 'simple instruction in drawing and painting' to members of the Navy, Army and Air Force 'to whom the other crafts made no appeal' which he expanded into a distinct practice categorised as art therapy.[65] The field was also developed in psychiatric hospitals, military medical hospitals and therapeutic communities as well as in art schools. Unlike the primarily diversional painting and drawing in asylums in the nineteenth and early twentieth centuries, art therapy posited art-making as a constitutively healing process. Many early pioneers were artists and pedagogues, like Hill, whose approaches were driven by convictions that art-making and art-viewing were intrinsically salubrious activities, rather than predicated on understanding of psychological mechanisms. The mentally healing function of art-making practices was often intertwined rhetorically with notions of art as broadly reparative and restorative, especially in the context of the Second World War when creativity was endorsed as being socially vital as a symbol of individual freedom.[66] The discourses of early art therapy often posited the nourishing and rejuvenating capacity of art. Arthur Segal, for example, another artist-pedagogue who pioneered art therapy in Britain in the late 1930s, claimed painting a 'life-giving source' that 'feeds and replenishes our individual selves with fresh energy'.[67] An émigré from Nazi Germany, Segal explored how painting could be used therapeutically at his Painting School for Professionals and Non-Professionals which he opened in London in 1937 with his wife Ernestine and daughter Marianne Segal. What differentiated Segal's approach practically at the time was that it centred not on painting imaginative subjects or articulating thoughts or emotions to cathartic effect but on representing external objects. He understood therapeutic effects to derive from methodical examination of the construction of three-dimensionality by light and shade. Students were led to paint naturalistic still-lifes and portraits by focusing on light, form and colour, an interest evident in Segal's own artworks after 1930, such as *Apples in a Bowl* (1938) (Fig. 10.3).

Psychotherapists referred patients to Segal's school, and the institution worked closely with an organisation called Q Camps which established an innovative therapeutic community camp called Hawkspur in rural Essex in 1936. Described as a self-governing educational community for young men aged between 16½ and 25 with 'behaviour problems' or who were 'unable to fit into normal society', Hawkspur pioneered 'planned environment therapy' which prefigured the post-war therapeutic community movement.[68] The camp regime itself was the holistic instrument of rehabilitation with responsibilities shared between members to facilitate democratic decision-making, self-discipline and social integration. There were in addition individual 'special treatments' which most commonly constituted regular psychotherapy but which for some members included attending Segal's painting classes. One young man went to the school regularly, the results of which were measured primarily in terms of his overall disposition, social adjustment and psychological and behavioural changes. The painting lessons led, according to one report, to 'marked improvement in all symptoms. [He] became articulate, intelligent in conversation, thoughtful, sensitive, industrious and much less unstable'.[69]

A critical site for power and agency in the history of art therapy is the interpretation and ownership of the objects made in this type of context. Analysis of artworks by therapists can disempower the maker since it implies, as art historian David Lomas notes, that 'without the intervention of the expert', the participant 'knows not what they say'.[70] Non-directive and non-interventionist approaches, prevalent in the 1950s, argued that the role of therapists was to facilitate rather than to direct

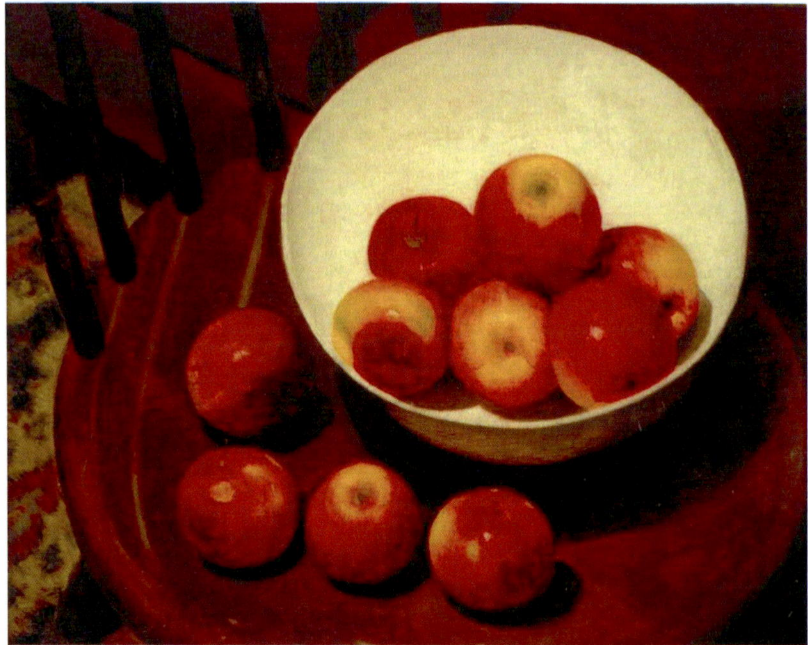

Fig. 10.3 *Apples in a Bowl*, 1938, Arthur Segal (1875–1944). Oil on panel, 39 × 50 cm. Guildhall Art Gallery, City of London Corporation.

practices and to interpret images. One of the most influential art therapists working in this vein was Edward Adamson who was appointed 'art master' at a long-stay psychiatric hospital at Netherne in Surrey in 1946. Initially Adamson was employed to contribute to psychiatric research into art as a means of treatment and diagnosis, whereby the patient-made works were analysed by doctors in clinical meetings. Adamson himself, however, emphatically rejected psychopathological and diagnostic readings of the works.[71] Once the original experiment had ended in 1951, he had greater autonomy and continued to run his non-interventionist art studio in the hospital's grounds until 1981, allowing residents to paint freely.[72] Having joined Netherne when lobotomies, electric shocks and insulin coma treatments were still widely used, Adamson conceived painting as individual and humane, operating in opposition to the hospital's institutional routine. His work constitutes a significant example of art practices being deployed to provide a critical mediation within an established mental-health treatment context.

The largest collection of art therapy works in Britain is the Adamson Collection, amassed at Netherne and now mostly housed at the Wellcome Collection (London). In line with the shift towards patient-orientated medical histories, artworks by patients, like those in the Adamson Collection, have been considered in recent years as valuable articulations of individual experiences that counter homogenising diagnosis-cure institutional histories of psychiatry.[73] The capacity of these objects to represent the voices of their marginalised makers is, however, fundamentally contingent on how they are treated and displayed contemporarily. In terms of the proprietary status of the objects, the Adamson Collection Trust (ACT) delineates its role not as the owner but the 'caretaker', 'rescuer' or 'guardian' of the works.[74] The decision has also been made, where possible, to name the makers of the artworks, as was the case in the exhibition *Mr A Moves in Mysterious Ways* (Peltz gallery, Birkbeck, University of London, 2017). Co-curator Fiona Johnstone argued that naming was essential in order to foreground 'individuals with their own personal histories' rather than a 'generic mass of psychiatric patients', a position informed by Richard Sandell that in a museum context 'anonymity can be construed as dehumanising'.[75] A point of comparison to this approach is a psychiatric 'objective scientific investigation' of the Prinzhorn collection that took place in 2017 which used modern art in public collections as 'control samples'. This 'computer-based analysis' compared 'schizophrenia' artworks with 'artworks by healthy artists' and found that images in the Prinzhorn collection by six of the fourteen artists selected possessed 'image properties that deviate from the range of values obtained for the control artworks'.[76] In this case, the possibility of reading the artworks as articulating the individual experiences and voices of those in asylums is curtailed by the study's pathological premise which implied from the start that the objects could reveal symptomatic formal properties. Ethical questions about ownership, naming and terminology are, crucially, not only historically embedded in the production of the work but are by necessity present-day concerns about how material should be read, displayed, interpreted and labelled responsibly. This is a key instance, then, of how probing mental-health care through the lens of its entanglement with art brings to the fore the importance of power and agency in histories of mental illness and treatment.

Conclusions

In conclusion, art was an arena in which practices, concepts and objects of mental-health care were not only circulated and shared but also interrogated and produced in the first half of the twentieth century. During this period, there was a fascination in the actual and imagined psychological effects of viewing and making art, conceptualisations of art became increasingly inflected at this time with issues pertaining to psychological health, while avant-garde artists seized on psychotherapeutic regimes as a means of creative inspiration and subversion. The discourses and practices of art not only supported but also challenged therapeutic routines: Adamson operated within a psychiatric institution but offered an influential intervention in its methods through his art studio. Surrealist artists mythologised and exploited mental illness, but aspects of their work can be understood to some extent as a cultural strand concerned, albeit problematically, with questioning psychiatric labels of 'normal'. This chapter has also shown that art was a centre for defining and creating healthy minds in a multitude of ways. The historically contingent instances of how viewing art by professional artists was perceived to contribute to mental well-being resonate with the well-recognised idea today that the visual arts and museums can play a role in supporting psychological welfare, particularly in the context of health being increasingly understood as a societal concern.[77] The incorporation of divergent visual and tactile art-making practices into a range of different therapeutic systems and institutional contexts in the newly emergent fields of occupational therapy and art therapy in the first half of the twentieth century attests to the varied positions of art within broadening mechanisms of prevention and remedy. Moreover, the fact that these therapeutic applications of art were driven by diverse ideas concerning the role of handicrafts, holistic concepts of the body and the nourishing and socially regenerative function of creativity, as opposed to models of the mind, evidences how psychological health has been directed by a broad set of discourses. Art informed and constituted methods of healing and shaped perceptions of mental illness both within the psychiatric institutions that are conventionally associated with treatment and outside in museum and pedagogic contexts that consequently formed part of the expanded terrain across which twentieth-century mental-health care operated.

Acknowledgements The author gratefully acknowledges the support of the Wellcome Trust and the University of Leicester, 204801/Z/16/Z.

Notes

1. Gemma Blackshaw, "The Pathological Body: Modernist Strategising in Egon Schiele's Self-Portraiture," *Oxford Art Journal* 30, no. 3 (2007): 377–401. See also Gemma Blackshaw and Leslie Topp, eds., *Madness and Modernity: Mental Illness and the Visual Arts in Vienna 1900* (Farnham: Lund Humphries, 2009).
2. Briony Fer, "The Role of Psychic Disorder in the Surrealist Aesthetic," in *Realism, Rationalism, Surrealism: Art Between the Wars*, eds. Briony Fer, David Batchelor, and Paul Wood (New Haven and London: Yale University Press in Association with Open University, 1993), 209–221; David Lomas, *The Haunted Self: Surrealism Psychoanalysis Subjectivity* (New Haven and London: Yale University Press, 2000), 53–65.
3. For a critical deconstruction of this narrative, see Griselda Pollock, "Artists, Mythologies and Media—Genius, Madness and Art History," *Screen* 21, no. 3 (1980): 57–96.
4. Emma Barker, Nick Webb, and Kim Woods, "Historical Introduction: The Idea of the Artist," in *The Changing Status of the Artist*, eds. Emma Barker, Nick Webb, and Kim Woods (New Haven and London: Yale University Press, 1999), 7–11. On the gendered construction of the artist, see Griselda Pollock and Rozsika Parker, *Old Mistresses: Women, Art and Ideology* (London: I.B. Tauris, 2013), 82–83.
5. Debora L. Silverman, *Art Nouveau in Fin-de-Siècle France: Politics Psychology and Style* (Berkeley: University of California Press, 1992).
6. Henri Matisse, "Notes d'un peintre," *La Grande Revue* 52 (25 December 1908): 731–45, reprinted in English in Jack D. Flam, *Matisse on Art* (London and New York: Phaidon, 1973), 38.
7. Joyce Henri Robinson, "'Hi Honey, I'm Home': Weary (Neurasthenic) Businessmen and the Formulation of a Serenely Modern Aesthetic," in *Not at Home: The Suppression of Domesticity in Modern Art and Architecture*, ed. Christopher Reed (London: Thames and Hudson, 1996), 98–112.
8. Robinson, "'Hi Honey, I'm Home,'" 101.
9. Roger-Ballu, *Exposition de Tableaux, Pastels, Dessins par M. Puvis de Chavannes* (Paris: Galerie Durand-Ruel, 1887), 7. Trans and cited in Robinson, "'Hi Honey, I'm Home,'" 108.
10. James Fox, *British Art and the First World War, 1914–1924* (Cambridge: Cambridge University Press, 2005), 127.
11. For this and the impact that theories of perception had on aesthetic theories, including Empathy Theory developed by Theodor Lipps and Adolf von Hildebrand, see Charlotte Klonk, "Patterns of Attention: From Shop Windows to Gallery Rooms in Early Twentieth-Century Berlin,"

Art History 28, no. 4 (2005): 468–496; Michael Hatt and Charlotte Klonk, *Art History: A Critical Introduction to Its Methods* (Manchester and New York: Manchester University Press, 2006), 66–90.

12. Klonk, "Patterns of Attention," 480.
13. Tanya Sheehan, *Doctored: The Medicine of Photography in Nineteenth-Century America* (University Park: Pennsylvania State University Press, 2011), 81–83. For a comprehensive history of different kinds of light therapies in Britain, see Tania Anne Woloshyn, *Soaking Up the Rays: Light Therapy and Visual Culture in Britain, c. 1890–1940* (Manchester: Manchester University Press, 2017).
14. Sheehan, *Doctored*, 82.
15. On Féré, see Christopher Turner, "Cured by colour," *Tate Etc.* 4 (Summer 2005); John Gage, *Colour and Meaning: Art, Science and Symbolism* (London: Thames and Hudson, 1999), 31–32. On chromotherapy, see R. Douglas Howat, *Elements of Chromotherapy: The Administration of Ultra-Violet, Infra-Red and Luminous Rays through Colour Filters* (London: Actinic Press, 1938).
16. James Fox, "Conflict and Consolation: British Art and the First World War, 1914–1919," *Art History* 36, no. 4 (2013): 810–833.
17. "The Influence of Colour," *The British Journal of Nursing* (7 September 1918): 153.
18. Fox, "Conflict and Consolation," 827.
19. Wassily Kandinsky, *On the Spiritual in Art* (1912) reprinted in *Kandinsky: Complete Writings on Art, Vol. 1*, eds. and trans. Kenneth C. Lindsay and Peter Vergo (London: Faber and Faber, 1982), 114–219.
20. On Kandinsky's approach, see Robin Veder, *Modern Art and the Economy of Energy* (Hanover, NH: Dartmouth College Press, 2015), 262–264.
21. For a discussion of how the artist considered abstract art to require changes in viewing habits, see Riccardo Marchi, "October 1912: Understanding Kandinsky's Art 'Indirectly' at Der Sturm," *Getty Research Journal* 1, no. 1 (2009): 53–74.
22. Adrian Stokes, "Form in Art: A Psychoanalytic Interpretation," *The Journal of Aesthetics and Art Criticism* 18, no. 2 (1959): 193–203.
23. See in particular Fer, "The Role of Psychic Disorder in the Surrealist Aesthetic," 212–218; Lomas, *The Haunted Self*, 53–65.
24. "Le cinquantenaire de l'hystérie, 1878–1928," *La Révolution Surréaliste*, no. 11 (1928). See Fer, "The Role of Psychic Disorder in the Surrealist Aesthetic," 212–218. On the cultural formations of hysteria see also Elisabeth Bronfen, *The Knotted Subject: Hysteria and Its Discontents* (Princeton, NJ: Princeton University Press, 2014).
25. "Le cinquantenaire de l'hystérie, 1878–1928," 20. Cited in Fer, "The Role of Psychic Disorder in the Surrealist Aesthetic," 212.

26. Antonin Artaud, *Van Gogh: The Man Suicided by Society* (1947) in *Antonin Artaud: Selected Writings*, ed. Susan Sontag (Berkeley and Los Angeles: University of California Press, 1998), 483–514.
27. André Breton, "Manifesto of Surrealism" (1924) in *Manifestoes of Surrealism*, eds. and trans. Richard Seaver and Helen R. Lane (Ann Arbor: University of Michigan Press, 1972), 5. On Ernst's image, see Lomas, *The Haunted Self*, 60–61.
28. Sander L. Gilman, *Difference and Pathology: Stereotypes of Sexuality, Race, and Madness* (Ithaca: Cornell University Press, 1985), 228–229.
29. Umberto Boccioni et al., "Futurist Painting: Technical Manifesto" (Italy: Poesia, 11 April 1910) reprinted in English in *Art in Theory, 1900–2000: An Anthology of Changing Ideas*, eds. Charles Harrison and Paul Wood (Oxford: Blackwell, 2003), 150–152.
30. Luke Heighton, "Josef Karl Rädler, *Untitled* (Self-Portrait), 1913," in *Madness and Modernity*, eds. Blackshaw and Topp, 110–117.
31. See *Beyond Reason: Art and Psychosis: Works from the Prinzhorn Collection* (London: Hayward Gallery, 1996); Catherine de Zegher, ed., *The Prinzhorn Collection: Traces Upon the Wunderblock* (New York: Drawing Center, 2000).
32. Anne E. Bowler, "Asylum Art: The Social Construction of an Aesthetic Category," in *Outsider Art: Contesting Boundaries in Contemporary Culture*, eds. Vera L. Zolberg and Joni Maya Cherbo (Cambridge: Cambridge University Press, 1997), 11–36.
33. See Hal Foster, "Blinded Insights: On the Modernist Reception of the Art of the Mentally Ill," *October* 97 (2001): 3–30.
34. Foster, "Blinded Insights," 3–4. See also Susan Hogan, *Healing Arts: The History of Art Therapy* (London: Jessica Kingsley Publishers, 2001), 57–61.
35. Catherine de Zegher, "A Subterranean Chapter of Twentieth-Century Art History," in *The Prinzhorn Collection*, ed. de Zegher, 3. On collections of 'insane' art, see John M. MacGregor, *The Discovery of the Art of the Insane* (Princeton, NJ: Princeton University Press, 1992). For a challenge to the dominant teleological narrative in which the 'art of the insane' became valued through Prinzhorn, see Allison Morehead, "The Musée de la folie: Collecting and Exhibiting chez les fous," *Journal of the History of Collections* 23, no. 1 (2011): 101–126.
36. Gilman, *Difference and Pathology*, 231.
37. Hal Foster, "Blinded Insights," 3.
38. The affinities that modern artists sought to suggest between their art and the 'art of the insane' were reaffirmed in the 1930s by the National Socialists under the umbrella of degeneracy. *Degenerate Art* exhibitions,

staged to ridicule modern art, drew explicit parallels between modernism and mental illness.

39. *Surrealist Objects and Poems* (London: London Gallery, 1937).
40. Alfred H. Barr, Jr., ed., *Fantastic Art, Dada, Surrealism* (New York: Museum of Modern Art, 1936), 12–13.
41. Barr, *Fantastic Art*, 13.
42. "Lettre aux médecins-chefs des asiles de fous", *La Révolution surrealiste*, no. 3 (15 April 1925): 29. Cited in Lomas, *The Haunted Self*, 60.
43. Lomas, *The Haunted Self*, 60.
44. See Imogen Wiltshire, "Therapeutic Art Concepts and Practices in Britain and the United States (1937–1946)" (PhD diss., University of Birmingham, 2017).
45. Alfred P. Solomon, "Rehabilitation: Opportunities for Psychotherapy in Physical Therapy," *Occupational Therapy and Rehabilitation*, no. 6 (December 1943): 286–293.
46. A. Rivett, "Fabric Printing," *Journal of the Occupational Therapists' Association* 1, no. 2 (October 1938): 19–22.
47. M. Jackson, "Weaving as a Curative Agent," *Journal of the Occupational Therapists' Association* 1, no. 1 (June 1938): 25–26.
48. Ana Carden-Coyne, "Ungrateful Bodies: Rehabilitation, Resistance and Disabled American Veterans of the First World War," *European Review of History: Revue européenne d'histoire* 14, no. 4 (December 2007): 543–565.
49. Virginia A. M. Quiroga, *Occupational Therapy: The First 30 Years 1900 to 1930* (Bethesda, MD: The American Occupational Therapy Association, 1995), 31.
50. Dorothea Robertson, "Occupational Department," *Annual Report of the Royal Glasgow Mental Hospital* (Glasgow Royal Asylum) (Glasgow: Glasgow Royal Asylum, 1923), Records of Gartnavel Royal Hospital, HB13/2/224, NHS Greater Glasgow and Clyde Archives, 29.
51. Annie H. Melrose, "Occupational Therapy Department," *Annual Report of the Royal Glasgow Mental Hospital* (Glasgow Royal Asylum) (Glasgow: Glasgow Royal Asylum, 1926), Records of Gartnavel Royal Hospital, HB13/2/224, NHS Greater Glasgow and Clyde Archives, 30.
52. "Scotland," *The Lancet* 203 (22 March 1924): 621.
53. Beth Linker, "The Business of Ethics: Gender, Medicine, and the Professional Codification of the American Physiotherapy Association, 1918–1935," *Journal of the History of Medicine and Allied Sciences* 60, no. 3 (2005): 320–354. See also Beth Linker, "Strength and Science: Gender, Physiotherapy, and Medicine in Early-Twentieth-Century America," *Journal of Women's History* 17, no. 3 (2005): 106–132.
54. Evelyn M. Carrington, "Psychological Foundation of Occupational Therapy," *Occupational Therapy and Rehabilitation*, no. 4 (August 1946): 141–144.

55. Quiroga, *Occupational Therapy*, 37–41.
56. See Quiroga, *Occupational Therapy*, 236–238; Elizabeth Casson, "The Prescription in Occupational Therapy," *Journal of the Occupational Therapists' Association* 1, no. 2 (October 1938): 22–24.
57. Ruth Ellen Levine, "The Influence of the Arts-and-Crafts Movement on the Professional Status of Occupational Therapy," *The American Journal of Occupational Therapy* 41, no. 4 (1987): 248–254. See also Quiroga, *Occupational Therapy*, 13–14.
58. Dorothea Robertson, "Occupational Department," *Annual Report of the Royal Glasgow Mental Hospital* (Glasgow Royal Asylum) (Glasgow: Glasgow Royal Asylum, 1924), Records of Gartnavel Royal Hospital, HB13/2/224, NHS Greater Glasgow and Clyde Archives, 26; Melrose, "Occupational Therapy Department," 32.
59. Joyce Hombersley, "Correspondence" (22 November 1944), *Journal of the Association of Occupational Therapists* 8, no. 21 (February 1945): 11.
60. Cited in Quiroga, *Occupational Therapy*, 236.
61. Ann Wilcock, *Occupational for Health, Vol. 2: A Journey from Prescription to Self-Health* (London: British Association of Occupational Therapists, 2002), 283–328.
62. See Hogan's survey history of art therapy in Britain, *Healing Arts*. For the USA, see Maxine Borowsky Junge, *The Modern History of Art Therapy in the United States* (Springfield, IL: Charles C. Thomas, 2010).
63. A key example is Melanie Klein, *Narrative of a Child Analysis: The Conduct of the Psycho-Analysis of Children as Seen in the Treatment of a Ten-Year Old Boy* (London: Hogarth Press and Institute of Psychoanalysis, 1961).
64. Erich Guttmann and Walter Maclay, "Clinical Observation on Schizophrenic Drawings," *British Journal of Medical Psychology* 16, nos. 3–4 (July 1937): 184–205.
65. Adrian Hill, *Art Versus Illness: A Story of Art Therapy* (London: Allen & Unwin, 1948), 26.
66. See Brian Foss, *War Paint: Art, War, State and Identity in Britain, 1939–1945* (New Haven and London: Yale University Press, 2007), 157–158.
67. Arthur Segal, "The Objective Principles of Painting," trans. Victor Grove, unpublished typescript (1929), Arthur Segal Collection, Box 1, Folder 17, Leo Baeck Institute, New York, 23.
68. Marjorie Franklin, ed., *Q Camp: An Epitome of Experiences at Hawkspur Camp (1936 to 1940) for Young Men Aged 16½ to 25* (London: Planned Environment Therapy Trust, 1966), 10. On Hawkspur in the context of therapeutic communities, see Tom Harrison, *Bion, Rickman, Foulkes, and the Northfield Experiments: Advancing on a Different Front* (London: Jessica Kingsley Publishers, 2000), 68–71.

69. Franklin, *Q Camp*, 48.
70. Hogan, *Healing Arts*, 15.
71. Susan Hogan, "British Art Therapy Pioneer Edward Adamson: A Non-interventionist Approach," *History of Psychiatry* 11, no. 43 (August 2000): 259–271.
72. See Hogan, *Healing Arts*, 169–80.
73. Alexandra Bacopoulos-Viau and Aude Fauvel, "The Patient's Turn Roy Porter and Psychiatry's Tales, Thirty Years On," *Medical History* 60, no. 1 (2016): 1–18.
74. David O'Flynn, Solomon Szekir-Papasavva, and Chloe Trainor, "Art, Power, and the Asylum: Adamson, Healing, and the Collection," *The Lancet Psychiatry* 5, no. 5 (May 2018): 369–399.
75. O'Flynn, Szekir-Papasavva, and Trainor, "Art, Power, and the Asylum," 398.
76. Gudrun Maria Henemann, Anselm Brachmann, and Christoph Redies, "Statistical Image Properties in Works from the Prinzhorn Collection of Artists with Schizophrenia," *Frontiers in Psychiatry* 8 (December 2017): 1–15.
77. Jocelyn Dodd and Ceri Jones, *Mind, Body, Spirit: How Museums Impact Health and Well-Being* (Leicester: Research Centre for Museums and Galleries [RCMG], University of Leicester, 2014), 3.

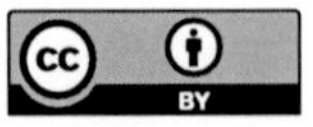

CHAPTER 11

The Myth of Dream-Hacking and 'Inner Space' in Science Fiction, 1948–2010

Rob Mayo

Introduction

Christopher Nolan's 2010 science fiction action film *Inception* was a commercial blockbuster, making back over five times its $160 million budget at the box office. It is also an enduring pop-culture reference point, parodied in episodes of *South Park* and *Rick and Morty*, and has even been recognised as the source of a neologism, with the suffix '-ception' becoming shorthand for the film's multi-layered plot. It remains one of the most memorable action films of the century due to the unorthodox setting of its heist plotline in the minds and dreams of its characters rather than in the film's real world, an aspect which has been more reverently carried by later television series such as *Sherlock* and *Legion*. As influential as it has become in contemporary culture, however, *Inception* is not the originator of this trope. Consciously or not, Nolan's film enters into a thematic tradition which had existed in Anglophone science fiction for over half a century before 2010. The trope of rendering a person's mind as a physical 'inner space' or landscape which can be explored

R. Mayo (✉)
University of Bristol, Bristol, UK
e-mail: rm13712@bristol.ac.uk

S. J. Taylor and A. Brumby (eds.), *Healthy Minds in the Twentieth Century*, Mental Health in Historical Perspective,
https://doi.org/10.1007/978-3-030-27275-3_11

and interacted with is therefore a kind of modern myth: creative works which adopt this theme reflect contemporary society's ideas and beliefs about how the mind works, how it may become damaged and how it may be fixed.

Like many other cultural tropes—superheroes, vampires or zombies, for example—'dream-hacking' fluctuates in popularity. Although this timeline begins with a short story from 1948, a small canon of inner space fiction first appears in the 1960s, among the writers whose work formed the 'new wave' movement in science fiction literature. One such author, J. G. Ballard, popularised the term 'inner space' in his critical writings and interviews, defining it as 'an imaginary realm in which on the one hand the outer world of reality, and on the other the inner world of the mind meet and merge'.[1] Typically this 'realm' is a virtual manifestation of 'the inner world of the mind' which does not 'meet' the outer world so much as co-opt properties of it. Aspects of outer-world physical space such as landscape, architecture and atmosphere thereby become metaphors for elements of intangible, ineffable mental experience. Ballard's concept of inner space is clearly reflected in the works of his contemporaries John Brunner and Roger Zelazny, which I consider alongside Peter Phillips's 1948 short story 'Dreams are Sacred' in the first part of this essay.

The second golden age of inner space fiction, examined in the second part of this essay, occurs in the 1980s. This period is one of diversification for the genre; the texts surveyed here include not only novels by Pat Cadigan and Greg Bear but also the first inner space film, *Dreamscape* (1984). Although still concerned in each case with exploring psychologically disordered minds, these texts each expand the potentials of inner space exploration beyond the asylum or psychiatrist's office; *Dreamscape*, for example, imagines the technology being co-opted by political conspirators, while *Mindplayers* (1987) imagines 'pathosfinding' as merely one service among many in a future world in which mind-altering technology is available recreationally. The final part of this essay examines inner space texts of the twenty-first century, which continue the trend established in the 1980s of moving from the page to the screen. In addition to *Inception*, I examine *The Cell* (2000), which covers ground later trodden by Nolan's blockbuster. I also explore the world(s) of *Psychonauts* (2006), a platform game directed by Tim Schafer, whose levels are each a virtual-physical representation of a character's mind. Although *Inception* is the end-point of the timeline traced here,

I conclude with a brief consideration of where the genre may go next, based on trends identified across the three sets of texts.

Before charting the course and future movements of inner space fiction, however, we may consider where it comes from.[2] Although 'Dreams are Sacred' is the starting point for this timeline, there are of course earlier texts that prefigure some generic elements. Many of the texts examined here contain echoes of psychomachia, the medieval genre of poetry and drama which includes the poem of the same name by Prudentius and the morality play *Everyman*. Although now readily associated with the mind, the prefix 'psycho-' derives from the ancient Greek word (*psukhē*) for 'spirit' or 'soul'. The concept of a conflict (*makhē*) in which the soul may be both the prize and the battleground may be seen, updated to refer to the mind instead of the soul, in many of these texts. Another early precursor is Leibniz's 'mill argument', which attempts to demonstrate the inviolable division between mental and physical phenomena. Leibniz asks his reader to:

> suppos[e] there were a machine, so constructed as to think, feel, and have perception, it might be conceived as increased in size, while keeping the same proportions, so that one might go into it as into a mill. That being so, we should, on examining its interior, find only parts which work upon one another, and never anything by which to explain a perception.[3]

Although Leibniz presents this as absurd, the image of someone 'enter[ing]' into a 'thinking machine' (i.e. a mind) and 'examining its interior' in order to infer its function recurs throughout these texts. Finally, the most immediate conceptual influence is of course psychoanalysis. The prevalence of 'dream-hacking' as the method of entering and exploring inner space is no doubt traceable to Freud's assertion that '[t]he interpretation of dreams is the [...] royal road to knowledge of the unconscious in the life of the mind'.[4] Even more fundamental to the genre, Freud's *oeuvre* provides a series of metaphorical models for the mind's functions, the most influential of which—conventionally known as Freud's 'topographical' and 'spatial' models—represent the mind as a varied and demarcated space (Figs. 11.1 and 11.2).

In Freudian accounts of the mind, there are strata of mental activity, with conscious thought elevated (or perhaps perched precariously) *above* a chaotic underworld of unconscious mental processes. This element of depth, which is common to both the topographical and spatial models,

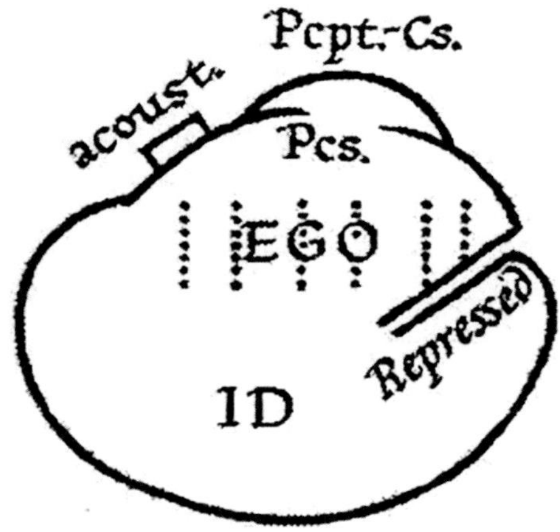

Fig. 11.1 A diagram of Freud's model of the mind in 'Ego and the Id' (1923). Public domain

is echoed in many of the texts examined in this essay. The influence of all of these precursors, from *Psychomachia* to Freud, is evident from the first inner space fiction.

1948–1966: The Emergence of a Genre

A relative unknown among the inner space authors surveyed here, Peter Phillipps produced a series of short stories between 1948 and 1958 before retiring from creative writing. 'Dreams are Sacred' was among the earliest and remains his best-known due to its origination of the dream-hacking trope. The anonymous protagonist/narrator is untrained in psychiatric medicine, but meets with 'a college friend [...] who'd majored in psychiatry' and is swiftly persuaded to enter 'the phantasmagoria of a brilliant mind driving itself into insanity through the sheer complexity of its own invention'.[5] The narrator is deemed capable of this due to both his professional distance and his 'cast-iron non-gullibility complex', and Phillipps makes much of the comic conflict between the patient, a pompous fantasy author and the narrator's deadpan 'iconoclastic manner'.[6] The technology facilitating this miracle is the encephalograph, used for its conventional purpose until 'one of [the doctor's] assistants stepped up the polarity-reversal of the field – that is, the frequency – by accident'.[7] Phillipps affords far greater attention to the possibilities of this technology than to the (pseudo)science behind it, and

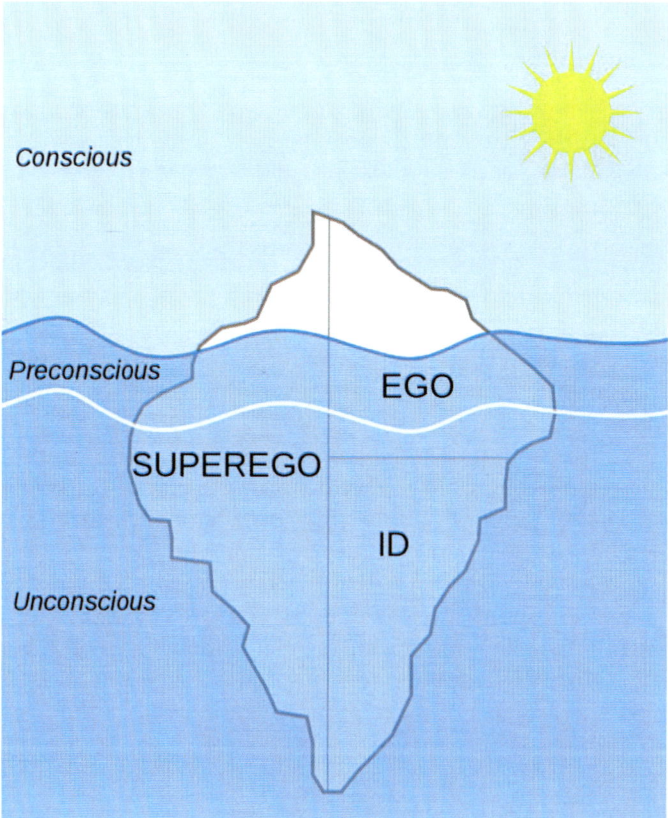

Fig. 11.2 Illustration of the iceberg metaphor commonly used for Freud's model. Public domain

the world of Marsham Craswell's mind vividly reflects his manic condition. The narrator initially finds himself in a desert landscape under two suns, surmising that 'this heat [is] generated by Craswell's imagination'. The blasted desert landscape is arguably a poor metaphor for Craswell's hyperactive mind, but the narrator's remark is telling; the atmosphere is 'generated by Craswell's imagination' in that he has imagined it, but it also recalls his doctor's diagnosis that his catatonic state is caused by his imagination operating in 'high gear' and suggests that this ambient heat is symptomatic.[8] The Citadel of the Snake provides a more visual metaphor:

> like a wedding cake designed by Dali, in red plastic:– ten stories high, each story [*sic*] a platter half a mile thick, each platter diminishing in size and offset on the one beneath so that the edifice spiralled towards the brassy sky.[9]

Craswell and the narrator continue on through many other imagined spaces, each reflecting Craswell's insanity through an environmental metaphor: 'the Hall of Madness, where strange music assaults the brain', for example, and 'a great, high-vaulted chamber [where the] lighting effects [...] were unusual and admirable – many colored shafts or radiance from unseen sources'.[10]

The narrator is immune to all danger while he is aware of the fantasy of his surroundings and, like a lucid dreamer, he can create allies and objects to help him survive. The only instance in which he is endangered is when he stops to consider 'whether the whole business was quite – decent', a momentary doubt which 'negates confidence. With confidence gone, the gateway is open to fear'.[11] The danger of the situation is not that any of Craswell's imagined perils might genuinely cause harm, but that the narrator might mistake the fantasy for reality and 'let [his] mind go under', which would result in him 'wak[ing] up as a candidate for a bed in the next ward'.[12] Although untrained in psychiatry, the narrator is evidently aware of Freudian theory and speculates firstly that '[Craswell's] affronted ego had assumed the whole power of his brain', and secondly that 'the death-urge [which is typically] buried deep, but potent, in the subconscious [...] was not buried deep here'.[13] This latter diagnosis suggests a territorial shift in the topography of the mind, with an element of the subconscious rising up to the conscious ego level, thereby taking over 'the whole power of his brain'. This image is also reflected in the virtual manifestation of the death-urge, '[a]n obscene hulking gob of animated, semi-transparent purple flesh' which looms over Craswell and the narrator once they arrive in 'the center of an enormous, steep-banked amphitheatre'.[14] Analogous to '[a]n ant in the bottom of a washbowl with a dog muffling at it', the spatial relation between the men and 'the Beast' also demonstrates the change that has occurred in the structure of Craswell's mind.[15]

Once the beast is defeated in psychomachia and Craswell's mind is returned to health, the story shifts to speculate on the wider significance of this technology, beyond the controlled psychiatric environment in which it is initially contained. The narrator discovers that characters summoned by him and Craswell to the dream world were not entirely artificial but drawn from their memories of the real world, and that real people have experienced strange dreams which reflect their roles in the story. The narrator and Dr. Blakiston conclude that the machine, unknown to them, 'became a transmitter'.[16] Contrary to the narrator's concern for the 'decency' of invading other minds, the story concludes with him ominously telling a young woman who rejects his romantic advances, 'I can wait. I'll be seeing you. Happy dreams'.[17] Phillipps's story thereby suggests that while the speculated technology may be valuably applied to treat mental disorder, it is liable to be abused if applied beyond the psychiatric world.

As Phillipps ended his literary career, many themes of 'Dreams are Sacred' were taken up in John Brunner's 1958 story 'City of the Tiger', which later formed part of his novel *The Telepathist* (1964; also published as *The Whole Man*, outside of the UK). As the UK title suggests, Brunner's fiction differs from Phillipps's in that telepathy—that is, communication between minds *without* technological broadcast—is a fundamental aspect of the plot throughout. Aside from a brief dalliance with organised crime before the protagonist, Gerald Howson, truly understands his abilities, the power of telepathy is primarily associated with psychiatry. The plot of the novel is structured around a series of missions undertaken by Howson, and his colleagues within a professional institution, to fix disordered minds. While following the psychiatric premise of its precursor, then, *The Telepathist* expands the application of dream-hacking to present several minds which are disordered in different ways. In the first mind which Howson explores, for example, the subject is a deaf-mute girl who is not intellectually disabled—'the lack was in the nerves connecting ears and brain, and in the form of her vocal cords'—but whose mental structures have nevertheless been uniquely shaped by her physical disabilities.[18] Exploring various 'areas' of her memories, Howson observes that 'because she had never developed verbal thinking [...] she used kinaesthetic and visual data in huge intermingled blocks, like a sour porridge with stones in it'.[19]

The spatial description is more explicit in later episodes, when Howson—now trained as a telepath—is tasked with extracting other telepaths from 'catapathic' states.[20] Echoing the premise of 'Dreams are Sacred', this occurs to telepaths who 'retreat into fugue and make a fantasy world which is more tolerable [than reality]'.[21] This is first demonstrated by Phranakis, a Greek general who avoids the consequences of defeat by creating a world, 'nurtured in his subconscious', where he is celebrated as a victor.[22] In contrast to the deaf-mute's—and indeed to 'the chaos of [the] subconscious' in a neurotypical, able-bodied character later—Phranakis's inner space is clearly figured as a recognisably human structure: 'Down the streets of his brain a procession moved [...] The city was safe'.[23] Ilse, the telepath who precedes Howson into this world, laments that Phranakis's secure mental city 'hasn't left *room* for intruders' and is overwhelmed by his mental defences which manifest as military guards.[24] Although it is a symptom of her peril rather than its cause, Ilse becomes 'uncertain where the illusion ended' as she is overwhelmed by Phranakis's mind, echoing Phillipps's story.[25] With Howson's assistance, Ilse escapes and completes her mission; Phranakis experiences extraction from his dreamworld as an image of 'the sky rolled back, like a slashed tent, and the gods were manifested'.[26] The imagery here clearly evokes his Greek heritage, but more subtly the spatial relation between Phranakis and the rupture in his inner space reflects his location in the Freudian *sub*conscious and his imminent upwards travel towards consciousness.

This first period culminates in the first iconic work of inner space fiction, Roger Zelazny's 1966 novel *The Dream Master* (a novella-length version, 'He Who Shapes', was published in *Amazing Stories* in 1965). Unlike 'Dreams are Sacred' and *The Telepathist*, which devote significant proportions of their total lengths to establishing the premise of inner space exploration and offering some explanation for its practice in their speculative worlds, Zelazny's novel begins *in media res* and only depicts the 'real' world after several pages. The novel's first inner space is a visually symbolic pastiche of Roman/Shakespearean history, as the protagonist Render ('the Shaper') partakes in the stabbing of Marcus Antonius while a perplexed Caesar looks on and protests 'I want to be assassinated too [...] It isn't fair!'.[27] This bizarre scene is explained when, in the real world, Render 'lift[s] off his crown of Medusa-hair leads and microminiature circuitry' which connects him to the 'ro-womb', an ovoid device containing his patient, Representative Erikson.[28] Like his precursors, Render is an uncommonly qualified 'neuroparticipant therapist', 'one of the two hundred or so special analysts whose own psychic makeup permitted them to enter into neurotic patterns without carrying away more than an esthetic gratification from the mimesis of aberrance:'; recalling 'Dreams are Sacred' particularly, Render's gift is his resistance to his patients' neuroses.[29]

In my reading of the Phranakis episode in *The Telepathist*, I identified visual symbolism which reflects the specific character and neuroses of the dreamer, and spatial imagery which calls to mind Freudian models of the mind which are theoretically common to every human mind. The opening scene of *The Dream Master* also displays this variation, as the assassination of Marcus Antonius reflects both the patient's real-world career as a senior politician and his baseless 'fears of assassination', while the 'darkness [...] constrict[ing]' at the 'periphery' of the dream appears to be an environmental manifestation of the sense that the dream is 'about to end'—that is, it is suggested to be inherent to the dream setting rather than particular to the dreamer.[30] Interpreting these metaphors, however, is complicated by the role of Render as the 'shaper' of the dream. Erikson protests that Render's interpretation of this dream is not really valid since his 'ability to make things happen stacks the deck', and Render confirms that he 'supplied the format and modified the forms'.[31] Render's ability to appear from behind 'a previously unnoticed corner' as a different character and then disappear 'around another sudden corner' is therefore not symbolic of Erikson's fragile hold on reality or the mental contortions required to maintain his paranoid fantasy, but simply a display of Render's directorial control over the dream.[32] Render clarifies that although he created the dreamspace it is Erikson who 'filled [it] with emotional significance, promoted [the events] to the status of symbols corresponding to [his] problem', and Erikson's concession that the dream had 'strong meaning' for him demonstrates that Render's diagnosis of Erikson is correct and that the visual symbolism is 'a valid analogue'.[33] The form of inner space explored in *The Dream Master* therefore corresponds to those of 'Dreams are Sacred' and *The Telepathist*, but with the new development that the psychiatrist's role is to craft a symbolic space which aids in their treatment of the patient, rather than searching for diagnostic clues or attempting to fix 'aberrance[s]' in a space which is created entirely by the patient's mind.[34]

Unlike *The Telepathist*, *The Dream Master* focuses on just one patient after Render concludes his business with Erikson. Dr. Eileen Shallot is another gifted psychiatrist, who seeks Render not for psychiatry but professional development; she is born blind and seeks to overcome this disability by training as a shaper. Render warns that her unfamiliarity with visual stimuli means that she must deal 'constantly [...] with the abnormal' when treating patients in this way, and that '[i]f the therapist loses the upper hand in an intense session he becomes the Shaped rather than the Shaper'.[35] This reasserts a didactic point connecting Phillipps's and Brunner's works, that immersion into another person's mind, particularly a disordered mind, entails the risk of annihilation. This common aspect of the inner space trope calls to mind both the classical mytheme of catabasis—the heroic descent into the underworld—and an inversion of the myth of Daedalus and Icarus: rather than flying too high and inevitably falling back down, the dream-hacker risks descending so far down into the mind that they are unable to emerge again. All of Howson's missions in *The Telepathist* end in success, and despite its pessimistic twist ending the inaugural inner space trip in 'Dreams are Sacred' concludes without harm to the protagonist. *The Dream Master*, in contrast, breaks new ground for the genre by depicting this disaster instead of merely suggesting its threat.

Ignoring his own counsel, and tempted by the prospect of pioneering work, Render agrees to give Eileen her first experience of sight by training her in neuroparticipation. The worlds which he creates for her are mundane, realistic environments, which is appropriate to Render's task of accustoming her to sight rather than of addressing a neurosis through symbolic tableaux. In their final session, Render creates from memory a cathedral but discovers that he is losing control and notices 'the altar [which he] had never seen before, anywhere [...] The organ chorded thunder under invisible hands'.[36] Panicking, he runs from Eileen and finds it to be 'like running through a waist-high snowdrift', and soon thereafter finds himself stood right next to Eileen again.[37] This image of motionless running recalls Erikson's feeling of having 'moved far from the circle of assassins, but the scene did not diminish in size', confirming Render's loss of control and new status as the 'shaped' rather than the shaper in Eileen's dream.[38] The scene of this final dream is either the lakeside cathedral conjured from Render's memory or the black void that remains when Render banishes his images, until he attempts to 'break the entire illusion' by refusing Eileen's amorous feelings.[39] Declaring his hatred of her transports him to a new space 'in the midst of a white plain. It was silent, it was endless. It sloped away towards the edges of the world'.[40] This blank, blasted landscape soon changes into a mutable and threatening world, quite unlike the controlled and everyday environments of his previous dreams with Eileen. Render is pursued by a monstrous wolf 'over crevasses and rifts, through valleys, past stalagmites and pinnacles – under the edges of glaciers, beside frozen riverbeds, and always downwards'.[41] This downward motion is emphasised by a change in Render's physical movements, as he runs 'through veils of snow which now seemed to be falling upward from off the ground – like strings of bubbles'.[42] As these snowflakes do indeed become bubbles, and Render's running motion is transformed into a headlong dive—'[l]ike a swimmer he approached'—it seems that this chaotic inner space alters to encourage his immersion in the chaotic Freudian subconscious.[43] Even after Render finds himself on solid ground again his downward motion is seemingly irresistible, as a 'chasm open[s] behind him' and he willingly topples into 'Vernichtung' ('annihilation'), bringing '[e]verything [...] to an end'.[44]

1981–1990: The Second Age of Inner Space

After the initial blossoming of the genre in the 1960s, inner space fiction seems to lose its appeal for SF writers for over a decade. The next author to take up the trope is Pat Cadigan, who in 1981 published the first of several stories featuring a protagonist named Deadpan Allie. These stories were reworked to form parts of her debut novel, *Mindplayers*. Although *Mindplayers* is predated by *Dreamscape*, I examine Cadigan's work first as many of her novel's depictions of inner space derive from the earlier stories.

Allie is introduced to the reader experiencing temporary and recreational psychosis using an illegal device called a 'madcap' which, like all other inner space directed devices in the novel, functions via electrical connections which go 'under [her] eyelids and around [her] eyeballs to the optic nerve'.[45] This brief introductory scene establishes that Allie is uninitiated and unqualified in psychiatric work, although when the authorities discover her 'unique brain organization' they decide to offer her employment, instead of a more punitive sentence, as a means for her to atone.[46] While Allie is therefore akin to the other protagonists examined so far, in that she accesses inner space by virtue of exceptional innate ability, *Mindplayers* presents a more egalitarian vision of the future in which the experience is available outside of the psychiatric institution. In this sense, *Mindplayers* is most like *The Telepathist*, and it also shares with it an episodic structure that depicts different minds through the exploration of inner space. Cadigan's first innovation is to begin this series with an image of Allie's own, healthy mind. Cadigan also considers the ethical implications of the technology—more thoroughly than 'Dreams are Sacred'—but Allie is eventually persuaded by her trainer that '[i]t's not going to be anything like rape [...] we'll meet in mind-to-mind contact. But I won't be *in* your mind'.[47] Having consented to the training, Allie finds herself at 'the edge of a broad field bounded by a low, flimsy wire fence; a roughly made sign [...] read[s] WATCH THIS SPACE'.[48] Since her trainer, Segretti, is also present here, it seems that this is the neutral space of 'the system' that he promised they would meet in, although Allie describes it as both her 'point of departure' and 'home'.[49] Less ambiguous is the cathedral which bears a sign stating 'YOU ARE HERE. And below, in smaller letters: WHERE DID YOU THINK YOU WERE?'; Allie identifies this simply as 'whatever area of [her] mind [she] was in', but the sarcastic sign suggests that this represents her ego.[50] Accordingly, Segretti is unable to join her when she ventures inside, in keeping with his promise that he could not enter inner space which is entirely hers. The cathedral, observed from outside, is constantly 'shifting and changing', presenting a pulsing mass of different architectural styles including 'traditionally Gothic' and 'log cabin'.[51] Inside Allie discovers a room, 'nothing like the interior of a cathedral', which contains an assemblage of significant objects and images from her life, 'things [she]'d owned or wished [she] had, souvenirs of things [she]'d done or seen'.[52] This TARDIS-like space suggests that Allie's sense of self is illusory; her ego is inconstant and diverse, and her understanding of herself as a coherent and constant persona is primarily based upon these memories.

This depiction of Allie's healthy mind is an ingenious contrast for those which she later explores as a 'pathosfinder'—one who, like a psychotherapist, searches for the causes of mental disorder. Her first assignment is Marty Oren, a reclusive actor whose mind initially manifests as 'a bare, sterile room [with] no windows, no doors, nothing, just smooth white walls'.[53] The contrast to the more pastoral scene in her own mind is striking, but Allie declares that the 'Infamous White Room' is a common phenomenon.[54] As she takes 'a walk through his life', however, this blank space is shown to be significantly apt.[55] This biographical exploration is manifested as 'a long hall lined with locked doors', which are discovered to be 'all empty. There was nothing to see in any of them and no sign of anything ever happening there'.[56] In contrast to Allie's cathedral, which contains vibrant reminders of her fondest memories, this corridor is 'just a space in [Marty's] mind. His body was an instrument rather than a live thing, his face a device [...] He just couldn't care'.[57] Allie does not definitively diagnose Marty—unlike Render, she does not typically employ a psychiatric discourse—but the contrast between his inner space and hers clearly suggests a lack of sense of self and connection to the world, akin to anhedonia or even psychopathy. Accordingly, when Marty attempts to exert control over the space and form a new landscape 'all he could manage was a bare earth under a colorless, sunless sky'.[58]

This dismal, barren space in turn provides an illuminating contrast with another space that Allie explores later, belonging to a schizophrenic poet. Kitta Wren's inner space is 'awash in lazy spiral rainbows and harlequin rivers', a fantastical and hallucinatory landscape. As in Marty's mind—and like Howson's exploration of the deaf-mute girl's memories—Allie experiences units of thought as physical objects, and 'move[s] in among a jumble of unfinished ideas' when she 'beg[ins] to get the feeling [she is]n't alone'.[59] Since Kitta is dead she is not present in her inner space, but Allie's intuition is verified by a manifestation of Kitta's psychosis, which strikes 'like a concentrated, highly localised storm'.[60] This functions in much the same way as a real-world storm, and Allie experiences it as 'the hard beat of the rain'.[61] However, it is of course also symbolic; the psychosis which ultimately drove Kitta to violent suicide is also credited with driving her career as a poet, as '[t]he seizure [tears] into her ideas and images and they scattered in all directions [...] a literal brainstorm [...] stirring her thoughts into new and better patterns'.[62] The notion of a connection between madness and creativity is a long-held one, but Cadigan innovatively imbues it here with a spatial aspect that depicts how sublimely terrifying the experience of a psychotic episode might be.

While Cadigan was publishing the stories that would eventually form *Mindplayers*, *The Dream Master* found a second life when inner space fiction made the leap from the page to the screen. *Dreamscape*, written by David Loughery and directed by Joseph Ruben, began as an outline written by Zelazny in 1981 based on his novel. The film stars several prestigious actors, including Max von Sydow and Christopher Plummer, but unfortunately lacks the impressive visual effects of contemporaneous SF films such as *Blade Runner* (1982) or *Aliens* (1986). While the film in general and its first two brief inner space scenes in particular have dated very badly, it deserves to be remembered for more than simply being the first inner space film.[63] Its climactic conflict is based around the question only alluded to in 'Dreams are Sacred'—what happens when this revolutionary technology, designed for psychotherapeutic use in a controlled medical environment, escapes the psychiatric institution? Although *Dreamscape* also briefly (and gracelessly) considers the potential for technology to be used for sexual manipulation, its core premise is that those killed in a dream die in real life, and so Plummer's machiavellian character plots to assassinate the US president.[64] Before discovering this, the protagonist Alex carries out psychiatric work to aid a child troubled by recurring nightmares. The boy's inner space is presented as a darkly lit house, which he anticipates will be invaded by a half-man, half-snake monster.[65] In an uncharacteristically artistic touch, this besieged domestic space is rendered with sharp and irregular angles, recalling the iconic sets of the German Expressionist classic *Das Cabinet des Dr. Caligari* (1920). When the monster strikes, Alex and the boy flee down a staircase which appears to descend endlessly and float in the middle of a black void.[66] Their panicked flight through twisting corridors at the eventual base of these stairs is accompanied by flickering overhead lights and several cuts from the camera filming them from behind to face-on, effectively conveying a sense of disorientation.[67] Their downward motion, recalling that of Render in *The Dream Master*, suggests a descent from a disordered ego/conscious deep into a chaotic and overwhelming id/subconscious. In accordance with much of Freud's theory regarding this model of the mind, it is in the subconscious that Alex and the boy can effect therapeutic change and kill the monster.

This stand-out set piece is in many ways recreated, with less visual flair, for the film's climactic psychomachia as Alex attempts to rescue the president from the assassin, Tommy.[68] The president's journey with Alex, pursued by Tommy, follows a familiar itinerary: they begin in an enclosed space (a train car instead of the boy's house); when a malevolent outsider arrives, they escape by moving downwards (a train station escalator instead of the floating staircase); they arrive at a dead end having descended as far as possible, and, as in the boy's dream, it is here that the dreamer can arm himself and kill his attacker, despite the apparent hopelessness of the situation. The president's subconscious space is even more chaotic and hostile than the boy's, as he and Alex are chased by red-eyed wolves which seem endemic to his mind rather than a manifestation of Tommy's assassination attempt, and the environment presents hazards in the form of loose electrical cables and rifts in the ground.[69] If, as the repeated set-piece elements suggest, this space should be interpreted as a physical manifestation of Freudian subconscious, then psychotherapeutic intervention is both necessary for the alleviation of mental disorder but also a distressing and dangerous experience.

A thoroughly more effective depiction of inner space is provided by Greg Bear's 1990 novel *Queen of Angels*, the final entrant in this middle period. The narrative is composed of four parallel plotlines emerging from a brutal mass murder carried out by Emmanuel Goldsmith. In one, a pioneering and 'O.V.F.&I. – Once Very Famous and Influential' psychiatrist, Martin Burke, is hired by the wealthy father of one of the murder victims to examine Goldsmith (and his inner space, or 'Country of the Mind') to try to discover the reason for the massacre.[70] Bear's speculative future reflects the passage of thirty-plus years since the publication of 'Dreams are Sacred'; the procedure is facilitated by a 'vial of nanomachines' mapping Goldsmith's brain, and the explorers interact with the world with the help of a 'toolkit [...] a simulated bright red box within which floated a display of circumstances of the probe', calling to mind the menu window of a video game.[71] Bear seemingly draw influence from Brunner, as Burke's declaration that '[i]n most of [his] previous incursions into the Country the central symbol of the mind had been a city' recalls the Phranakis episode in *The Telepathist*.[72] Of course, this violent murderer's inner space is unlike Burke's previous patients', even though the medical and psychological tests carried out on Goldsmith by Burke's team prior to the procedure show that '[w]ithin certain limits [his] brain and body functions are normal'.[73] Burke observes that Goldsmith uses '[n]o personal pronouns at all' when discussing the murders, a tic which he (mis)construes as evasion of responsibility.[74]

The chapter depicting Burke's and his colleague Carol Neuman's journey into Goldsmith's mind is a narrative *tour de force*, and perhaps the most sustained depiction of a mental landscape in fiction. Recalling Render's fateful expedition at the end of *The Dream Master*, Goldsmith's inner space becomes chaotic, hostile and surreal, and Neuman is incapacitated; although she regains consciousness by the novel's coda, she and Goldsmith seemingly bear psychic scars from their traumatic experience. In contrast to the Brunner-esque inner spaces previously encountered by Burke, Goldsmith's mind initially manifests as 'torrid blue sky and endless desert', mysteriously concealing Goldsmith's 'deeper psychological processes' which Burke expects to be laid bare.[75] Instead of Freud's 'royal road to [...] the unconscious', they follow an 'excruciating[ly]' monotonous highway which abruptly ends at 'a vast canyon'.[76] In place of a city, there is 'a crystal-lined pit, the crystals resolving into buildings'.[77] This submerged/inverted city presents an unprecedented degree of 'contraction and desolation', which variously suggests '[a] pathology like the shrinking of tissue', 'major mental dysfunction', and 'internal genocide'—and, indeed, an erasure of the ego which Goldsmith's verbal tic suggested.[78]

Although *Queens of Angels* is unique among these texts in that the (living) person whose mind forms the landscape does not appear within it, Goldsmith's mind is not entirely uninhabited. Burke and Neuman anticipate 'figures symbolising Goldsmith's subpersonalities, his major mental organons, [who] would use speech', an idea which recurs in *Inception*.[79] There should also be 'a vivid population' in Goldsmith's city, comprising his memories of everyone that he has encountered in his life.[80] When Burke and Neuman arrive at the city centre, however, they discover a ghostlike population, among which 'the inhabitants [have] very little real individuality'.[81] Descending 'down several flights of stone steps' into an analogue of Grand Central Station—or, perhaps, into the anticipated 'deeper psychological processes'—they find a nightmarish scene of figures jumping to their deaths, the mounting corpses dangling from the cables on which they land.[82] As with the scene composed by Render for Erikson at the start of *The Dream Master*, this symbolic image defies and distorts physical distance, as Burke and Neuman perceive the corpses with 'nauseating conviction' and 'visual acuity [...] as if they were only a few meters away'.[83] Burke reassures Neuman that 'space [is] a true fiction' here, but spectral figures from Goldsmith's mind soon intercept and overwhelm them, demonstrating the truth of his prediction that 'being in direct connection with Goldsmith's mental symbology could conceivably disturb their own interior landscapes'.[84]

2000–2010: The Breakthrough of a Genre

The success of *Inception* marks the transition of inner space fiction from a marginal genre (SF literature) to a viable mainstream (Hollywood cinema). I have so far traced the development of the inner space trope throughout the mid-to late twentieth century and demonstrated that precursors to Nolan's film exist, mostly in literature. However, although it has greater cultural impact than all of these texts, *Inception* is not even the first inner space fiction of the twenty-first century. This most recent age was inaugurated instead by *The Cell*, another Hollywood film directed by Tarsem Singh. It begins, like *The Dream Master* and, later, *Inception*, in an inner space rather than in the real world, a distinction suggested almost immediately by the surreal transformation of Catherine Deane's horse into a two-dimensional replica after she dismounts.[85] This desert space is where she meets a boy whom she attempts to persuade to go sailing. The boy's resistance to this is reflected by the ships that he creates (and, arguably, by the desert setting in general); the first is a dilapidated tanker half buried in the sank, the second a small toy boat. After the boy runs away in anger, his and Deane's bodies are shown suspended by a mysterious machine, revealing that this shared simulation is part of a therapeutic attempt to extract the boy from a coma caused by a rare form of schizophrenia.

Deane's journeys into this space bookend the film's main narrative, which follows *Queen of Angels*'s lead; Carl Rudolph Stargher is a serial killer who is rendered comatose by the same disease, and whose latest victim is trapped in a hidden lair. Although she and her team are wary of exploring such a mind, Deane consents in order to find clues to the location of Stargher's victim. Singh's visual flair is most effectively deployed in the scenes of Deane's first venture, beginning with a sequence that represents her experience of being transported into Stargher's mind.[86] Singh cuts from Deane's eye to a close-up of the cloth covering her face for the procedure, zooming into and through an opening in the embroidery. The camera then rises out of a pond to reveal the baptism of a child, maintaining focus on the scene as the camera loops over and, now upside-down, submerges again on the other side. The unorthodox camera motion here suggests that incursion into another's mind requires first a transcendence of one's own inner space and secondly a disorienting re-submergence. This remarkable shot is followed by a continuing pan as the camera re-emerges in what appears to be a sewer. Maintaining the theme of disorientation—and reflecting, perhaps, the drastic recalibration that one might have to undergo in experiencing a mind like Stargher's—Deane is revealed lying unconscious on the left hand 'wall', the camera finally turning anti-clockwise to match her gravity. This perspectival trick is repeated on Deane's later excursion, when she awakes in a glass box on top of a stone tower.[87] As she pushes on the ceiling of the box it opens and she falls out, upwards, the gravity in Stargher's mind having suddenly changed as the box opens.

Stargher's inner space is not simply deceptive but atmospheric and dangerous. Although *Dreamscape* and *Inception* feature intertextual visual references, to *Das Cabinet des Dr. Caligari* and the Penrose steps (popularised by M. C. Escher), respectively, Singh demonstrates a far greater familiarity with visual art. Scenes set in Stargher's mind recreate visual artworks by H. R. Giger, Damien Hirst, and Odd Nerdrum, all of which are tonally appropriate for the dark atmosphere of Stargher's mind.[88] These are not simply tableaux but spaces which Deane and Special Agent Peter Novak must navigate: this is particularly evident in the scene in which Deane must walk between the glass sheets dividing the sections of a freshly dissected horse. This scene also emphasises the mechanical aspect of Stargher's mind, echoing Liebniz's depiction of the mind as a mill which one might enter. After passing through the horse Deane finds a room full of glass screens, where she ill-advisedly pulls a lever and presses a button.[89] Singh's camera jumps from mechanism to mechanism, showing the consequences of Deane's actions in a Leibnizian inspection that she regrettably neglects.

Deane's teammate warns that going 'very deep into [Stargher's] world' entails the risk of '[coming] to believe that [his] world is real [and] theoretically her mind could convince her body that anything that was done to it there is actually done'.[90] Continuous with the premise of *Dreamscape*, this means that '[if] you die in your dream, you die in real life'.[91] Deane demonstrates this by being overwhelmed by Stargher's mind and is rescued by Novak. *The Cell* breaks from generic tradition, however, in introducing the concept of 'reversal', in which the mentally disordered individual is brought into the therapist's mind instead of vice versa.[92] This ploy extracts Stargher's 'king' persona from his 'very twisted kingdom' and allows Deane to kill him; although this does indeed kill Stargher in the real world, along with the innocent child persona in his mind, this is presented as a redemptive moment for them both.[93] Recalling her enthusiasm to attempt reversal on her first patient at the start of the film, in order to 'show him a different place' from his own 'world which is not healthy' (i.e. his isolated mind), the film concludes with Deane and the boy in a space which merges aspects of both of their inner spaces (Deane's cherry trees blossom in the boy's desert landscape).[94] Here, Deane successfully simulates a sailing trip with the toy boat and a billowing blue cloth, suggesting the imminent success of her therapeutic strategy.

Just as inner space fiction first appeared in cinema in the 1980s, another significant jump to a new medium occurs in the twenty-first century. *Psychonauts*, a computer game developed by designer Tim Schafer and released in 2005, exploits the video game form to provide vibrant new explorations of inner space. The player controls Raz, a young boy attending a psychonauts training camp for children. The psychonauts gain access to minds using a small door (or 'portal') that they attach to people's heads. Although the leaders of the camp are depicted as adventuring spies—an application of inner space technology which anticipates *Inception*—the context of the game is often psychiatric, particularly in later levels based on the minds of people encountered in an abandoned mental asylum. (This is the only asylum depicted in these texts, and it is tellingly dilapidated and hazardous.) *Psychonauts* uses a variety of video game genres, but is primarily a platformer, a genre which involves traversing hazardous landscapes. Like many platformers since (and including) *Mario Bros* (1983), *Psychonauts* features collectible items. In the case of *Mario Bros*, these were coins, which could earn the player more lives. In *Psychonauts* the collectibles—figments of imagination, mental cobwebs, emotional baggage and mental vaults—have more thematic than functional value, although the vaults contain slideshows which reveal hidden information about the character whose mind is explored. These are often off of the path that the player needs to take to complete the level, suggesting that these memories are those that a character would rather forget and as such are kept remote spaces of the mind. One particularly effective instance of this is a whole hidden room which is impossible to access on the first pass through one of the psychonaut trainers' minds. More powerful abilities gained later provide access a room containing writhing demonic figures trapped behind a fiery barrier; read alongside information from Milla's mental vaults, one may infer that this hidden space represents the traumatic memory of surviving a fire in which the other children at her orphanage died.[95]

The use of space in other levels is even more sophisticated, if less dark. Another early level, in the mind of Milla's fellow trainer, Sasha Nein, is simply a large cube, reflecting Sasha's reserved nature and ostensible self-control.[96] The training exercise undertaken here leads to the explosion of material and adversaries from various faces of the cube; the material's emergence from below and formation in the shape of a crib or other items from Sasha's childhood present a visual depiction of Freud's notion of repression. (The player's task of sealing these ruptures suggests that Freudian repression is a natural process and not always unhealthy.) Even in the most chaotic moments of this level, the centre of gravity is always at the center of the cube; if Raz walks over the edge of the cube, that edge becomes the floor, so the danger of falling to one's death which is so common in platformer games is negated here. This is quite unlike the game's most disordered mind, which Raz encounters later at the asylum. Boyd Cooper is a security guard for the asylum but is overwhelmed by his obsession with conspiracy theories. On first entrance to his mind, this is visually depicted by the interior of Boyd's home, which features stereotypical newspaper cuttings and scrawls of handwriting on the walls.[97] This is the sanest area of Boyd's mind though—given the presence of Boyd himself there, perhaps this represents the ego—as leaving the house reveals a suburban street which twists and floats in a turquoise void. The polar opposite of Sasha's well-adjusted mind, this level exaggerates the generic threat of falling; the street not only features gaps that Raz must jump over, but its twists and turns mean that the gravity is not consistent: gravity always pulls Raz towards the pavement, but an adjacent street might be at a 90° angle to another, meaning that Raz must jump *at* it rather than across *to* it. As with the sequence introducing Stargher's mind in *The Cell*, the disorientingly inconsistent gravity reflects the disruption of a formerly normal, healthy mind, and the difficulty and dangers of exploring it.

Finally, the release of *Inception* in 2010 brings this latest phase of inner space fiction—and this timeline—to an end. Cobb and Arthur are 'extractors', corporate spies employed to steal information from business competitors' minds. A powerful businessman, Saito, employs them to perform 'inception', i.e. implanting an idea in someone's mind rather than extracting information, in the hope of convincing his rival, Fischer, to dissolve his late father's business empire. Not only does *Inception* imagine inner space technology applied to a novel purpose, it also presents the only speculative future in which the technology is truly separate from psychiatric institutions; Arthur states that 'the military developed dream sharing. It was a training program for soldiers to shoot, stab and strangle each other and then wake up', and the only passing allusion to psychiatry is Eames's facetious suggestion that the team should charge both Saito and Fischer for their services, given the catharsis that they induce pertaining to Fischer's strained relationship with his father.[98] In service of the corporate espionage theme and the heist-like plot of the film, *Inception* follows the example of *Psychonauts* and frequently includes vaults and safes in dreams, which Cobb says 'the mind automatically fills [...] with information it's trying to protect'.[99] In the same scene Cobb explains that '[y]ou can literally talk to my subconscious. That's one of the ways we extract information from the subject'.[100] Although this is a minor element of the plot, this strategy is more success for Cobb's team than Burke's and Neuman's interaction with Goldsmith's 'organons' in *Queen of Angels*.

Inception's greatest innovation is its nested narrative structure. When Arthur protests to Saito that inception is impossible Cobb insists 'you just have to go deep enough', and this is achieved not by a physical descent (as in the submerged city in *Queen of Angels*, or the staircases of *Dreamscape*) but by repeating the process of entering a shared dream state while already within a dream.[101] In one of the opening sequences, Cobb and Arthur attempt to steal secrets from Saito, and it is established that—in contrast to *Dreamscape* and *The Cell*—dying in a dream merely wakes the sleeper up. However, the mission into Fischer's mind requires them to descend three levels of dreaming, which necessitates a powerful sedative whose side effect is that anyone who dies will instead go to limbo, which is 'just raw, infinite subconscious', i.e. a wasteland filled with the ruins of buildings created by Cobb and his dead wife Mal when they previously ventured there.[102] It is from this biographical detail that the film derives its emotional core, and its hidden link to the psychiatric background of inner space fiction. Mal appears in any dream that Cobb inhabits, as his psychic projection of her is so powerful that it manifests and sabotages his mission by killing Fischer, sending him to limbo before he can open the vault in the final dream level. After Ariadne first encounters Mal while training in a dream with Cobb, she warns Arthur that 'Cobb has some serious problems that he's tried to bury down there', in a 'prison of memories' which is physically manifested in Cobb's dream as a lift shaft, with the scene of Mal's suicide kept on the basement floor: as in Freud's schema of the mind, repressed content is submerged deep in the subconscious, and like Freudian psychotherapy the speculative dream technology allows access to this.[103] By encountering Mal in limbo while rescuing Fischer and rejecting her appeals to stay with her, Cobb perhaps achieves catharsis and relief from his guilt over her death. If, as the film implies, both he and Fischer achieve a therapeutic benefit as a side effect of the heist, then *Inception* seems to join 'Dreams are Sacred' in suggesting that the depths of psychiatric probing required to relieve neurosis entail dangerous risks to all involved.

Conclusions: 'Which Way to Inner Space?' (J. G. Ballard, 1962)

I have traced the development of inner space fiction here among various media and across over sixty years, from 'Dreams are Sacred' in 1948 to *Inception* in 2010. Like many cultural tropes, inner space has experienced bursts of popularity—in the 1960s, then the 1980s, and finally, the first decade of the twenty-first century—and comparative absence from popular culture in the years in between. In the interests of covering sixty years in the space of an essay, I have limited the scope of study to anglophone SF texts and selected texts which I deem most germane or significant in the three periods examined. This regrettably entails the omission of non-anglophone texts such as Satoshi Kon's 2006 animated film *Paprika* (or the original 1996 novel by Yasutaka Tsutsui), texts by more mainstream authors such as Doris Lessing and Will Self, or SF texts which fit less comfortably into Ballard's definition of inner space, such as *Clans of the Alphane Moon* by Philip K. Dick. The readings that I have provided here highlight elements of continuity and diversity in these texts' conceptualisations of psychiatry and mental health through the theme of inner space, but not exhaustively. It is hoped that each of these texts and more may receive further attention through this critical lens, thereby furthering our understanding of the texts themselves, inner space fiction as a whole, and contemporaneous psychiatric thought.

From this sample, however, some clear observations emerge. The repeated appeal of the genre attests to a consistent desire on the audience's part to see the mind—an ineffable and ethereal realm, in the prevailing philosophy of Cartesian dualism—rendered in physical form. This desire is catered to by a shared symbology of spaces: landscapes, architecture and atmosphere, which attempt to translate the private experience of thought into terms more typically used to describe the physical world which we share. The texts examined here are also evidence of a lasting interest in mental disorder, as the genre typically depicts psychotherapists, or other characters whose minds are implicitly healthy, experiencing an explicitly disordered mind as a space which they must explore and interact with in order to provide therapeutic treatment. I suggest that this trope constitutes a modern myth not simply because it recurs in different media and time periods but because it frequently serves a didactic purpose. Some of the moral questions or lessons which connect many of the texts studied here, across the three time periods, include: the ethical propriety of attaining access to another person's private thoughts; the potential misuses of such a technology should it be removed from the psychiatric institution, and the notion that exploring another person's mind—particularly a mentally ill person's—entails a risk to the health of the explorer's own mind. The genre is, in this sense, frequently pessimistic; the idea of exploring another person's mind is consistently appealing, but the texts examined here often punish their protagonists for this transgression against natural order. The trope therefore echoes the classical myths of Prometheus or Icarus, who are each punished for their hubris. Conversely, however, several of these texts offer optimistic images of their protagonists overcoming the adversity of inner space and cultivating healthy minds, particularly those of the twenty-first century such as *The Cell*.

Scientific understandings of the material brain have advanced significantly since 1948, but unless and until neuroscience can account for all mental phenomena it seems likely that the concept of the mind and the symbology developed across these texts will retain their cultural currency. It has now been almost a decade since *Inception* was released which, according to the pattern established by this timeline, suggests that another surge of popularity for the genre may be imminent. It is perhaps also due to appear in a new media, given the jump to cinema in the 1980s and the transition to platformer computer games with *Psychonauts* in 2004. A sequel to *Psychonauts* is (at time of writing) planned for release this year, and a short single-episode connecting the two games, *Psychonauts in the Rhombus of Ruin*, was released for Playstation VR (a virtual reality video game headset) in 2017. Although it does not feature any inner space exploration, this highlights an intriguing possibility for the genre's future. If the symbology of the mind developed in SF texts since 1948 is rendered in the format of a virtual reality adventure game, inner space may in a sense become reality, allowing players to experience immersive worlds which, through landscape, architecture, and atmosphere, attempt to communicate the experience of mental disorder. Perhaps, despite a frequently reactionary tone throughout its history, inner space fiction may thereby conceivably come to have a practical therapeutic application.

Notes

1. J. G. Ballard, "Interview with J. G. Ballard," *Munich Round Up* (100), 106.
2. Except for *Inception*, the texts examined here have received scant critical attention. My primary aim in this essay is to establish an overview of the development of a narrative trope across various media in recent history;

I am therefore concerned less with situating these texts in the context of their (generally meagre) critical reception than with the conceptual context from which the idea of inner space derives.

3. Gottfried Wilhelm Leibniz, *The Monadology and Other Philosophical Writings*, trans. Robert Latta (London: Oxford University Press, 1898; reprinted in 1968), 228.
4. Sigmund Freud, *Interpreting Dreams*, trans. J. A. Underwood (London: Penguin Books, 2006), 623.
5. Peter Phillipps, "Dreams are Sacred," *Astounding Science Fiction*, September 1948, 53.
6. Phillipps, "Dreams", 55.
7. Ibid., 55.
8. Ibid., 53.
9. Ibid., 59.
10. Ibid., 61, 63.
11. Ibid., 65.
12. Ibid., 55.
13. Ibid., 65.
14. Ibid., 66.
15. Ibid.
16. Ibid., 69.
17. Ibid., 70.
18. John Brunner, *The Telepathist* (Harmondsworth: Penguin Books, 1968), 43.
19. Ibid., 43–44.
20. Ibid., 65.
21. Ibid., 66.
22. Ibid., 78.
23. Ibid., 75, 109.
24. Ibid., 78.
25. Ibid., 81.
26. Ibid., 86.
27. Roger Zelazny, *The Dream Master* (New York, NY: ibooks, 2001), 10, 12.
28. Ibid., 13–14.
29. Ibid., 22, 31.
30. Ibid., 9, 16.
31. Ibid., 15.
32. Ibid., 11–12.
33. Ibid., 15, 19.
34. Ibid., 22.
35. Ibid., 47.
36. Ibid., 240.

37. Ibid., 242.
38. Ibid., 11.
39. Ibid., 244.
40. Ibid.
41. Ibid., 245–246.
42. Ibid., 246.
43. Ibid.
44. Ibid., 250.
45. Pat Cadigan, *Mindplayers* (London: Gollancz, 1988; reprinted in 1989), 3–4.
46. Ibid., 17.
47. Ibid., 16.
48. Ibid., 21.
49. Ibid., 16, 21, 23.
50. Ibid., 25.
51. Ibid., 26.
52. Ibid.
53. Ibid., 130.
54. Ibid.
55. Ibid., 131.
56. Ibid., 132.
57. Ibid., 133.
58. Ibid.
59. Ibid., 165.
60. Ibid.
61. Ibid., 167.
62. Ibid., 166.
63. Joseph Ruben, dir. *Dreamscape*. Twentieth Century Fox, 1984. These scenes occur at 28 minutes and 18 seconds, and 40 minutes and 10 seconds.
64. Ibid., 58:04.
65. Ibid., 45:58.
66. Ibid., 47:26.
67. Ibid., 47:46.
68. Ibid., 1:22:42.
69. Ibid., 1:27:07.
70. Greg Bear, *Queen of Angels* (London: Gollancz, 1990; reprinted in 2010), 12, 14.
71. Ibid., 204, 271.
72. Ibid., 273.
73. Ibid., 204.
74. Ibid.

75. Ibid., 272.
76. Ibid., 274–275.
77. Ibid., 276.
78. Ibid., 278, 280.
79. Ibid., 277.
80. Ibid., 282.
81. Ibid., 281.
82. Ibid., 272, 282.
83. Ibid., 283.
84. Ibid., 275, 284.
85. Tarsem Singh, dir. *The Cell.* New Line Cinema, 2000. 1 minute and 19 seconds.
86. Ibid., 40:32.
87. Ibid., 58:09.
88. Ibid., 42:45; 44:12; 1:11:28.
89. Ibid., 45:26.
90. Ibid., 48:32.
91. Ibid., 48:53.
92. Ibid., 1:37:47.
93. Ibid., 51:42; 1:35:00.
94. Ibid., 11:03; 1:39:16.
95. Tim Schafer, dir. *Psychonauts.* Majesco Entertainment, 2004. This space appears in the 'Milla's Dance Party' level.
96. Schafer, *Pyschonauts*, 'Sasha's Shooting Gallery'.
97. Schafer, *Pyschonauts*, 'Milkman Conspiracy'.
98. Christopher Nolan, dir. *Inception.* Warner Bros. Pictures, 2010. The quotation appears at 27 minutes and 15 seconds; Eames's remark at 1:21:06.
99. Ibid., 28:18.
100. Ibid., 28:08.
101. Ibid., 20:54.
102. Ibid., 1:05:55.
103. Ibid., 33:00; 58:10.

Index

S. J. Taylor and A. Brumby (eds.), *Healthy Minds in the Twentieth Century*, Mental Health in Historical Perspective,
https://doi.org/10.1007/978-3-030-27275-3

W

Z

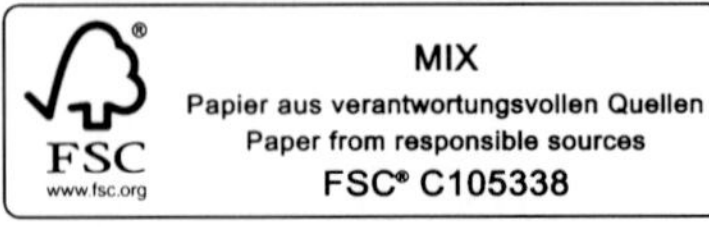

Printed by Books on Demand, Germany